'This long overdue volume of Margaret Rustin's legendary clarity of mind and thought. As has been the case for a very long time, Margaret is the "go to" person for an opinion or consultation; this book allows us to "find our way", in perpetuity, to her wise counsel.'

Ricky Emanuel, *child, adolescent and adult psychotherapist, London*

'Margaret Rustin's enquiring mind and her emotional receptivity are in constant dialogue in her endeavour to find a way to the child. Thanks to her unique capacity to connect the dimensions of her patients' external reality and their internal objects, and her organic integration of clinical experience and psychoanalytic theory, this book is a precious guide for practitioners, teachers and future generations of child psychotherapists.'

Suzanne Maiello, *child, adolescent and adult psychotherapist, Rome*

'This is a marvellous book. It is also a book of critical importance at a time when children's emotional health is a growing concern in this confusing and rapidly changing world. Margaret Rustin is a gifted writer and an unusually gifted psychoanalytic psychotherapist. *Finding a Way to the Child* is a compelling description of her work with children and adolescents over many years at the Tavistock Clinic. Rustin's vivid and detailed examples of trying to understand in depth the experience of each of her young patients and of finding ways, based on her exploration of psychoanalytic technique, of communicating that understanding in the most helpful way, includes also her examination of the doubts, distress and confusion that she needs to contain. The author understands that life is often difficult for babies and young children, even those raised in the most favourable conditions. Many of the children she sees have some difficulty in their background: illness or death in the family, loss of their national home, racial problems, extreme financial problems, adoption or being taken into care, etc. Some may have no obvious cause of their distress. The second half of the book, about assessment for treatment, deals with how decisions are made about which children will get treatment in this environment of limited resources. Rustin describes the great care that must be taken over these sometimes agonizing decisions, so that even when further treatment can't be offered, the child, and often the parents, can find the assessment process therapeutic in itself. Rustin's rich, detailed and clear presentations of her life's work will be of immense interest and help to colleagues in her own and related fields, experienced professionals and beginners alike; and, indeed, to anyone interested in children's emotional lives.'

Priscilla Roth, *British Psychoanalytical Society, London*

Finding a Way to the Child

Margaret Rustin's writing is characterised not only by its subject matter, which is diverse, but by her imaginative sensitivity to the emotional lives of children and young people, the depth of her understanding, and her original insights into the complexities of child and adolescent psychotherapy.

Here a selection of her work, edited by Kate Stratton and Simon Cregeen, is brought together in a collection which focuses mainly on clinical issues and concerns: the dynamics of the interaction between patient and therapist in the consulting room; the task of assessment; the particular needs of children and young people whose early development has been distorted by trauma, loss or neglect; and the framework and skills required for effective psychoanalytic work with parents. Illustrated by vivid narratives detailing the strains and possibilities of the therapeutic encounter, this book is a record of clinical work and thinking over 50 years of psychoanalytic practice.

It will prove essential reading for psychoanalysts and child analysts, child psychotherapists, all those training as mental health professionals in work with children and parents, and anyone with an interest in deepening their understanding of the emotional lives of children and young people.

Margaret Rustin is a child and adolescent psychotherapist and child analyst. She was head of Child Psychotherapy at the Tavistock Clinic 1985–2009 and played a major role in the extension of child psychotherapy training across the UK. Since retiring from the NHS, she has a private practice and teaches in many different countries. She has edited and written widely, most recently, jointly with her husband Michael, *Reading Klein*.

Kate Stratton is a child and adolescent psychotherapist in the Adolescent & Young Adult Service at the Tavistock Clinic where she also teaches and supervises. She is a former editor of the *Journal of Child Psychotherapy*, and co-editor of the Tavistock Clinic Series.

Simon Cregeen is a child and adolescent psychotherapist and couple psychoanalytic psychotherapist in independent practice. He teaches and supervises and has published in the *Journal of Child Psychotherapy* and elsewhere. He is a co-author of *Short-Term Psychoanalytic Psychotherapy with Adolescents with Depression: A Treatment Manual* (2016). He is a Trustee of Manchester Psychoanalytic Development Trust (mpdt.org.uk).

THE NEW LIBRARY OF PSYCHOANALYSIS
General Editor: Anne Patterson

The *New Library of Psychoanalysis* is published by Routledge Mental Health in association with the *Institute of Psychoanalysis*, London.
The purpose of the book series is:

- to advance and disseminate ideas in psychoanalysis amongst those working in psychoanalysis, psychotherapy and related fields
- to facilitate a greater and more widespread appreciation of psychoanalysis in the general book-reading public
- to provide a forum for increasing mutual understanding between psychoanalysts and those in other disciplines
- to facilitate communication between different traditions and cultures within psychoanalysis, making some of the work of continental and other non-English speaking analysts more readily available to English-speaking readers, and increasing the interchange of ideas between British and American analysts.

The *New Library of Psychoanalysis* published its first book in 1987 under the editorship of David Tuckett, who was followed by Elizabeth Bott Spillius, Susan Budd, Dana Birksted-Breen and Alessandra Lemma. The Editors, including the current Editor, Anne Patterson, have been assisted by a considerable number of Associate Editors and readers from a range of countries and psychoanalytic traditions. The present Associate Editors are Susanne Calice, Katalin Lanczi and Anna Streeruwitz.

Under the guidance of Foreign Rights Editors, a considerable number of the *New Library* books have been published abroad, particularly in Brazil, Germany, France, Italy, Peru, Spain and Japan. The *New Library of Psychoanalysis* has also translated and published several books by continental psychoanalysts and plans to continue the policy of publishing books that express as clearly as possible a variety of psychoanalytic points of view. The *New Library of Psychoanalysis* has published books representing all three schools of thought in British psychoanalysis, including a particularly important work edited by Pearl King and Riccardo Steiner, *The Freud-Klein*

Controversies 1941–45, expounding the intellectual and organisational controversies that developed in the British Psychoanalytical Society between Kleinian, Viennese and 'middle group' analysts during the Second World War.

The *New Library of Psychoanalysis* aims for excellence in psychoanalytic publishing. Submitted manuscripts are rigorously peer-reviewed in order to ensure high standards of scholarship, clinical communications, and writing.

For a full list of all the titles in the New Library of Psychoanalysis main series as well as both the New Library of Psychoanalysis 'Teaching Series' and 'Beyond the Couch' subseries, please visit the Routledge website.

Finding a Way to the Child

Selected Clinical Papers 1983–2021

Margaret Rustin
Edited by Kate Stratton and Simon Cregeen

Routledge
Taylor & Francis Group

LONDON AND NEW YORK

Cover image: Sphere with Inner Form, Dame Barbara Hepworth, 1963
Photo © Bowness

First published 2023
by Routledge
4 Park Square, Milton Park, Abingdon, Oxon OX14 4RN

and by Routledge
605 Third Avenue, New York, NY 10158

Routledge is an imprint of the Taylor & Francis Group, an informa business

British Library Cataloguing-in-Publication Data
A catalogue record for this book is available from the British Library

ISBN: 978-1-032-35153-7 (hbk)
ISBN: 978-1-032-35156-8 (pbk)
ISBN: 978-1-003-32554-3 (ebk)

DOI: 10.4324/9781003325543

Typeset in Bembo
by Apex Covantage, LLC

For Michael, and with thanks to the children, young people and families who have enabled me to do this work.

Contents

Author preface

My discovery of psychoanalysis and where it has led me

I was introduced to psychoanalysis during my university years through friends, when I was studying classics, and then, more formally, by my teachers during my subsequent philosophy degree. At this time I often felt that literature, politics or history were perhaps where my real interests lay. The remarkable thing over the years since then has been to realise that all these strands could come together meaningfully in my work as a child and later also an adult psychotherapist, and be further explored in my teaching and writing. Some of these connections are very evident in my writing, but not all are represented in this book with its presentation of clinical papers from my 50 years of practice.

In a second planned volume, the focus will be on the central role of infant observation in my psychoanalytic perspective, my contributions to the development of theory, some reflections on the experience of teaching, and the challenges of clinically relevant research in psychotherapy. Thus my abiding interest in a psychoanalytic exploration of literature, and in children's literature in particular, which has been pursued mainly in joint publications with my husband Michael Rustin, is not included here.

I began a personal analysis very soon after I completed my philosophy degree, and just as I was exploring my career direction. Was I to follow the academic path, or was my growing interest in psychoanalysis to lead me to seek to pursue clinical training? These early adult years had also been very turbulent ones, as they so often are, and I had little idea just how fundamentally my life would be reshaped by my analysis. The discovery of how very hard it was to think about oneself in an authentic way was a painful shock to me, as it overturned many assumptions I had had about myself and my world. It was overwhelming to be faced with the at times impossibly disparate tasks of embracing one's own emotional realities and also learning to look at and reflect on what one found. My privileged academic background had in no way prepared me for the struggle to integrate feeling and thinking, despite my belonging to a generation of young women who believed that there were vital connections between our personal experiences and the structures of social life and the way we understood ourselves.

The years of analysis encompassed not only my first experiences of working with young children (as a teacher of a group of a group of five and six-year-olds who could not be managed in their classrooms) and my intense years of training as a child psychotherapist, but also my first pregnancy, the birth of a daughter, and my early years as a mother. The good fortune of having an opportunity to have an analysis at this critical point of young adult life left me with a great interest in times of transition in life, from school to university and beyond, and in the beginnings of the lives of babies and their parents. It also shaped new forms of friendship, changed ideas about the meaning of political commitment, and offered me a quite new conception of what I wanted to do with my life, which was now to have the exploration of psychoanalysis at its heart.

Alongside my analysis, and integrally connected to it, was my outstanding educational experience of training as a child psychotherapist in this as yet tiny profession. I was rather dazzled by the insightfulness of my clinical supervisors at the Tavistock who included Martha Harris, Shirley Hoxter, and Esther Bick, and I was lucky to be part of a terrific group of fellow trainees from all over the world all of whom turned out to have a lifelong devotion to psychoanalysis. When I joined the Tavistock staff after qualification, I became part of a close group of child psychotherapy colleagues who shared a common culture linking together the practice of clinical child analysis to a commitment to improving public access to analytic therapy for children. The Tavistock I joined enabled child psychotherapy to grow and later become recognised as a new profession within the NHS, as Bowlby, Winnicott, and many in the analytic community had hoped when they supported its first steps in post-war Britain.

What I wish to emphasise is the profound impact made on me by what I saw as the privilege of undertaking clinical work with children and adolescents. The gift of analytic access to the unconscious structures of the mind to which my analyst had introduced me was now experienced from a new vertex. Encountering the inner lives of my child and adolescent patients, and the concreteness of unconscious phantasy as expressed in the relationships they made with me, led to an awed realisation of the immense potential for development which rested in the transference relationship. This gripped me, as no other work ever had done.

Psychoanalytic work with children and families keeps one close to the ongoing everyday intercourse of internal lives and external context. My pre-clinical work with children in a school had already alerted me to the way in which analytic ideas made sense of ordinary encounters, including one memorable day on which I was taking a little group of children on an outing by car. Imagine my shock to hear them lustily shouting out of the windows at the passing cars: "Missionary pigs!" Obviously this epithet belonged in truth to one view they had of me and my companion on this trip.

Despite my philosophical education and quite extensive reading of psychoanalytic literature both before and during my training, I really got to grips with psychoanalytic theory primarily in the consulting room. I found out in a particular way why Melanie Klein placed so much emphasis on the baby's relationship to the feeding mother and its aggressive dimension when one very disturbed little girl told me, as she clutched her face in her hands: "The bottle has bitten my nose off". Similarly I learnt what W. R. Bion meant by bizarre objects when studying the extraordinary drawings of another child and listening to her verbal confections. She had a whole private language which referred to what we would call part objects, in which she joined them together to form idiosyncratic shapes which were the stuff of her ongoing waking nightmares. The opportunity to work with severely psychotic young children was particularly important to me. What I came to realise, as wise supervisors had warned me, was that they would not recover to become 'normal', but that analysis did offer a chance for them to feel more human, and for their lives to become less dominated by terror and more open to friendly feelings and companionship with others.

The Tavistock public health context, in which such long-term clinical work over many years was supported and in which I was so lucky to work, also required us to give attention to preventive community work. Baby clinics, nurseries, play centres, schools, children's homes, youth clubs, and so on were the terrain of our efforts to support the understanding of children's developmental needs. All this provided a rich context for exploring the wider relevance of ideas which had their origin in the consulting room. Both in direct consultative work with professionals with many different roles in children's lives and in contributing to training courses of different kinds I found a deep connection to my experience in the playroom.

The richness of London's psychoanalytic culture in the second half of the twentieth century was the vital background to developments taking place at the Tavistock. I benefitted from a wealth of seminars and conferences as well as individual supervision and close professional friendships. Later in my career, it was also an honour to be invited to become an Honorary Associate of the British Psychoanalytical Society and to be recognised as a child analyst. This represented to me an acknowledgement of the inter-dependence of the home of psychoanalysis in Britain and its growing offshoot, the practice and profession of child psychotherapy.

I have been the recipient of much institutional and personal generosity over my more than 50 years as a child psychotherapist. Much of my writing has been in response to invitations to speak at conferences and to teach in different countries and continents. To give book-shape to very varied clinical interests was a challenge. The sections which emerged have been organised to foreground some of the long-term cases which meant most to me, to discuss issues of assessment in child psychotherapy, to represent my particular interest in children brought up outside their birth families, and to argue strongly for the importance of work with the parents who seek help for their children.

I hope the papers gathered here, which my thoughtful and patient editors have helped me to select and organise, will serve to represent my thanks for all the opportunities I have been given to learn and will also convey the remarkable ways in which psychoanalysis enriches our world.

INTRODUCTION

Simon Cregeen

Margaret Rustin is a psychoanalytic clinician, thinker, teacher, supervisor, and writer known internationally for her important contributions to the development of child and adolescent psychotherapy. During a clinical career that goes back over 50 years, she has written a great many papers, all of which convey her imaginative sensitivity to the emotional lives of children, young people and their families, and the depth and complexity of her understanding. They also demonstrate her insight into the intricate relationship between internal and external realities, and the social and political contexts for individual distress.

This is the first of two books gathering together some of Rustin's most significant papers. This volume is primarily dedicated to clinical papers and concerns and illuminates her commitment to close observation in the tradition of the psychoanalytic method. The second book will focus on infant observation, psychoanalytic theory, research, and supervision. Some of these papers have appeared in a variety of journals and books, and some have been revised for these volumes; others, originally presented at conferences and symposia, have not been previously published. Needless to say, a difficult part of this endeavour has been the selection of which papers to include and which to leave out. Notable omissions include the numerous articles she has co-written with others, including one important strand of her work – her writings, with her husband Michael Rustin, on children's fiction and drama. She has found deep sources of stimulation in literature throughout her career and although these papers are not included here, her understanding of the role imagination plays in

DOI: 10.4324/9781003325543-1

achieving emotional growth permeates all her writing, as does her analytic creativity and absorption in the lives of her young patients.

Reading through her papers, one is struck not only by the clarity of her thinking but also by the breadth of her areas of interest and associated publications. To bring serious-minded, high-quality attention to bear on such diverse concerns – from the internal object relations of the most troubled child to the political and social realities of human lives – is a rare gift, and we are fortunate to be able to benefit from the range contained in this book and the one to be published subsequently. Rustin's work is firmly located in the Kleinian tradition with its deep conviction in the power of unconscious phantasy, in the psychic reality lived within the transference relationship, and the centrality of close observation and working through in the countertransference. The substratum of this is a belief that all of us have a primary need to be known and to know others (Bion, 1962a).

The Tavistock Clinic and the NHS public service context

Rustin's writing draws upon a professional lifetime of clinical work with children, adolescents, and parents, primarily within the National Health Service (UK); her organisational home for more than 50 years was the Tavistock Clinic. The clinical work described in the following papers was undertaken primarily within this context. As many readers will know, the NHS was established in 1948 as a nationwide free service at the point of use, accessible to all, from cradle to grave. As an already established mental health organisation based on public service principles, the Tavistock Clinic became part of the NHS from its inception.

Rustin first arrived at the Tavistock as a child psychotherapy trainee in 1967, in one of the early cohorts when Martha Harris, a child and adult psychoanalyst who had trained under Esther Bick, was head of training. Harris was a significant influence upon Rustin's early development as a clinician and psychoanalytic thinker. As a student in her seminars, Rustin recalls how, 'we felt ourselves very fully known to her through these seminars but also to trust her use of this knowledge because it was used with love and concern to facilitate our development as individuals and as potential therapists' (1987). Writing of Harris's qualities, Rustin notes how

democratic instincts, personal generosity, a capacity for phenomenal hard work, and a conviction that the unique value of psychoanalytic insight ought to be shared as much as was possible
enabled Mattie (Martha Harris) to inspire her psychotherapist
colleagues to take on this challenge.

(ibid.)

Such a description could equally be made of Rustin's work and of
her commitment to the development of psychoanalytic ideas and
practice.

Following in the footsteps of her gifted teacher, in 1986 she took
on the responsibility of leading the child psychotherapy training at
the Tavistock, a role in which she remained until 2007; she continued as head of the child psychotherapy discipline at the Tavistock
until her retirement from the NHS in 2009. Rustin was an inspiring
presence at the Tavistock, making significant contributions to many
organisational developments within the wider clinical and training
environment. One of many examples was the introduction of the
Masters and later the Doctoral programmes into the framework of
the child psychotherapy training. The formal bringing together of
the clinical and academic created a solid base for child psychotherapists to develop their interest and confidence in clinical and conceptual writing for publication, and to pursue research interests within
an organised academic structure.

This has led to a flowering of academic papers and books which
describe the rich variety of child psychoanalytic work, and through
rigorous research studies, provide an evidence base for its effectiveness. In her co-editing of books bringing together a range of authors
and clinicians, and behind the scenes in situations where her name
doesn't appear, Rustin has helped many child psychotherapists to
develop their ideas and to write about their clinical experiences, and
encouraged them to publish. She believes passionately in the need
for the child psychoanalytic community to share their thinking and
practice, and sees writing as a vital aspect of analytic work, a way to
learn from others, and to interrogate the validity of one's ideas.

During Rustin's tenure, the Tavistock child psychotherapy training saw many more trainees coming from outside of London, thus
building the profession across the regions of the UK. Her experience
of growing up in the North of England is reflected in her enduring
commitment to the growth of psychoanalytic ideas and practice in

places far from the established heartlands of North London, and she has been involved in many training initiatives and study events in all four nations of the UK. One substantial and enduring example arose from her support for a proposal to establish an NHS training school in the North of England to train child and adolescent psychotherapists. In 2003 the Northern School of Child and Adolescent Psychotherapy, based in Leeds, took in its first cohort of trainees. This followed similar initiatives in Birmingham and Scotland. Rustin's encouragement and support has been profoundly formative for generations of child psychotherapists in the UK, and for others seeking to develop work with children and families in many other countries.

Writing

Rustin's clinical, theoretical, and research interests range far and wide. Her commitment to training child psychotherapists and to the broader development of the Tavistock has perhaps mitigated against developing a singular area of specialism. She views her range of interests as reflecting the many occasions on which she would find herself faced with a request: as she puts it, 'a paper or presentation or initiative was required and I would think, well somebody has got to do it!' So her attention was subjects and tasks to which she wouldn't otherwise have found her way. Rustin's pragmatic – and typically modest – view suggests her polymathy was simply born out of necessity. However, this underplays the depth of her clinical acuity and her unusual ability to bring psychoanalytic thinking to bear on disparate subjects.

What has been consistent is her lifelong devotion to investigating the ways in which psychoanalytic thinking and technique can significantly help the growth of mind and personality in children and young people whose early development has been distorted by trauma, loss, or neglect. Many of the papers presented here vividly demonstrate how Rustin enables her patients to begin to tolerate their emotional reality, to be known by another, and to become curious about themselves.

Research

Over the last 20 years there has been a rapidly developing interest in researching what it is that child psychoanalytic clinicians do and why some approaches seem particularly effective in bringing about personality growth and relationship change. With a shared commitment to the idea that psychoanalysis, since Freud, has always been a research programme located in the context of its clinical practice, Margaret and Michael Rustin have been central to this burgeoning research activity, not least as Clinical Doctorate supervisors to many research projects.

Michael's work as Professor of Sociology (University of East London) led to research models familiar within the social sciences being applied in child psychoanalytic research (Rustin & Rustin, 2019). The coupling of qualitative research models with psychoanalytic observational methods and clinical work has resulted in a rapidly growing child psychotherapy research literature, and an increased confidence within the profession about its value.

The pressing need to understand which treatments most help the increasing numbers of depressed adolescents led to a significant randomised control trial, the 'gold standard' in empirical research, to which Margaret Rustin made a major contribution. The Improving Mood with Psychoanalytic and Cognitive Therapies study (Goodyer *et al.*, 2017) included a manualised time-limited psychoanalytic intervention (Cregeen *et al.*, 2017) and resulted in the introduction of time-limited psychoanalytic treatment for depressed adolescents into the National Institute for Clinical Excellence (UK) guidelines. This was an important outcome and supported Rustin's longstanding belief that empirical research into psychoanalytic treatments is essential in order to strengthen the position of psychoanalytic psychotherapies within public health services.

Clinical perspectives

I would like to highlight a few examples from this collection of papers which demonstrate Rustin's particular integration of open-minded curiosity, clinical creativity, and responsiveness to the countertransference. It is worth noting that many of her patients were seen non-intensively (one or two sessions per week), as is the case for so many NHS patients seen by child psychotherapists. The clinical examples in her papers attest to the often-overlooked potential of such non-intensive psychoanalytic work. As will be evident from the following chapters, the location of the Tavistock Clinic in central London means that the range of patients and families seeking help is wide and inclusive. The diversity of cultures, ethnicities, sexualities, and familial structures is evident in Rustin's clinical papers, which cover a period of over 30 years.

It is sometimes suggested that Kleinian thinking and practice places insufficient emphasis on the external world and an individual's lived experiences. Contrary to this view, Rustin's clinical papers clearly show her belief that social, economic, and political realities play a significant role in the shaping of emotional life, an individual's sense of identity and belonging, and the nature of the internalised family culture. An individual's development may be promoted or hindered by these realities. The relationship between internal and external reality is a dynamic one and in constant flux, at its best stimulating creative development of inner life and the taking up of opportunities in the external world, and at its worst leading to despairing and destructive identifications and ways of relating to self and others.

This interaction is clearly illustrated in the first chapter in Section 1, 'Finding out where and who one is – the special complexity of migration for adolescents'. Here Rustin navigates the terrain of adolescent development, exploring the difficulties that arise when external life has been life-threatening and disorganised, and when there has been too early an exposure to dangers both physical and emotional. She shows how for young people with such life experiences, the ordinary processes of individuation in the context of adolescent development, and the achievement of a secure sense of self can become unmanageable.

In this chapter, Rustin focuses on the loss or absence of a sense of home for two patients, Vorjat and Wayne. Although their external life circumstances and deprivations were different, both boys were seriously depressed and struggling to develop a secure sense of belonging. Rustin explores how Vorjat, an asylum-seeking refugee from the Balkans living with his devastated family in the UK, and Wayne, an Afro-Caribbean boy who had been abandoned by his mother and was living in foster care, had been left psychically homeless, with little sense of the differentiation between internal and external worlds.

Rustin notes the powerful countertransference experiences aroused by clinical work with these two adolescents and the startling degree to which she was dependent on her own thoughts and feelings during long silences and absences from sessions. She is open about those moments in which her containing capacity fails and minor enactments occur, showing how when these can be considered with curiosity, rather than felt in a persecutory way, the meaning of what it was that was so difficult to contain may begin to be understood.

In the description of this work, Rustin's experience of loneliness, her difficulty in helping her patients to locate more negative feelings towards her, and her need to tolerate their helplessness are captured with evocative honesty. In reading the chapter, one feels for the adolescents, and one feels for the therapist. This chapter powerfully articulates how, with patients who have suffered as Vorjat and Wayne had, the therapist's task involves the bearing of the unbearable, what Bion termed 'nameless dread' (1962a). Rustin suggests that 'if it can be named, it is defused of some of its power and can then be further investigated, become an object of thought'.

In Section 2, Rustin's writings attend to the complex art of assessment. She emphasises the importance of considering the individual child's difficulties in the context of their experience of family life, along with the nature of their internal phantasies, their anxieties, and the ways they have sought to manage these. In 'Finding a way to the child', Rustin describes the process of her assessment of Alex, a troubled six-year-old boy living with a mother who was determined to get the necessary help for her son despite her own difficulties. At the point of referral, Alex was speaking of 'wanting to die, saying he would use a knife, and also sleepwalking'.

The chapter provides a single case example of Rustin's approach to assessment, the framework she provides for this, and the sensitivity with which she finds her way into the child's psychic reality. The account of the assessment sessions reveals her imaginative capacity to take in and recognise her young patient's fear, and Alex's experience of being trapped in it without respite or companionship. Using the toy figures, Alex begins 'an intricate non-stop game' where 'smaller and larger boys [are] fighting throughout, with murderous intent and great viciousness'. Jealousy and rivalry are present, and the play conveys a chaotic, terrifying, and relentless situation in which cruelty and violence are endlessly enacted.

The therapist's initial comments and enquiries about his play seem not to reach Alex, preoccupied as he is with the raw matter of survival. Rustin describes how at this point in the session she reviewed her own situation and found she was witness to an interminable horror story. Death was no end, since the protagonists were continually dying but immediately leaping to their feet and carrying on. . . . The barrage of torture, pain, hatred and fear was increasing and no framework of meaning which could make sense of why any of this was happening could be grasped.

This first assessment session, however, seems to bring Alex some relief and in the second session he is able to think and communicate more symbolically. He draws, plays, and talks to his therapist about his state of mind, providing 'a very vivid enactment of his experience of being deeply stuck in all these preoccupations and in despair about being able to free himself . . . the overall impression grew of a quite deathly and timeless stasis'. Rustin describes how she is struck by Alex's increased capacity to communicate once he has gained some sense of the clinic as a place offering help and containment. She feels this provides indications of his suitability for psychotherapy.

Section 3 focuses on Rustin's sustained interest in childhood deprivation and loss and includes writings about psychotherapy with children and young people who have early life experiences of abuse, abandonment, and dislocation. In the chapter 'Psychoanalytic work with an adopted child with a history of early abuse and neglect', Rustin writes about her work with a little boy, Tim, whose early life experiences and identification with damaged internal objects had created a way of relating dominated by 'ruthlessness and inaccessibility'. She describes how this was needed to protect him since the underlying situation was one of almost skinless vulnerability.

Rustin recounts how in the early period of work, 'there were many sessions which brought me to the edge of my capacities as a therapist', and describes how Tim would repeatedly leave her feeling 'lost and homeless in my room. I experienced shame and helplessness, knowing that he would jeer at whatever I said, and felt huge and foolish'. Tim's sense of worthlessness, terror, profound vulnerability, and his feelings of being psychically unplaced, thus painfully known in his therapist's countertransference, become the basis of Rustin's understanding of his primitive anxieties and necessary defences, and of the emotional qualities of his object relationships.

Over time there is a movement from absorbing the shock of frank aggression and standing up to Tim's tyranny to tender receptiveness to his infantile helplessness. Rustin's conviction about the importance of carrying on talking tells us about her deeply intuitive sense of what Tim needed at an infantile level in order to feel held and contained; her soft voice and words wrapping around him enable the development of a psychic skin. It is also characteristic of her belief in the importance of being able to put words to primitive emotional experience.

In her discussion of this clinical work, Rustin draws our attention to the concepts she is relying on, including Klein's view that the infant's anxieties arise 'not only from the fact of initial total dependence but also from the urgent pressure to be relieved of the terror aroused by his own overwhelming impulses'. Rustin goes on to refer to Bion and his theory of mind and pre-verbal communication. The clinical material describing her work with Tim illustrates how her conceptual framework supports her clinical approach in an unobtrusive way. The integration of theory and practice is deeply convincing.

The final Section 4 is concerned with working with parents. The analytic framework and skills required for effective psychoanalytic work with parents, who are usually not the 'referred patient', is a particular and enduring interest for Rustin. Her thinking in this area has adapted and developed over the years in response to changing societal conceptions of parents and parenting, and a plethora of parenting programmes within the child mental health field. Rustin's writing has made a significant contribution to the way in which work with parents and carers is conceptualised, underlining the vital contribution it can make, whether undertaken in parallel with the child or adolescent's therapy, or as a standalone treatment.

Rustin suggests that there are four main categories of work with parents. She goes on to describe her understanding of the aims and parameters of each of these areas of work, offering a sort of schema, not to be used as a route map but so that the delineated areas can be referred to as reference points to aid one's stance. This is a dynamic model where there can be movement and development between the four areas of work. Rustin suggests that any shift from one domain of work to another needs to be made explicit, and that 'signalling this can both give us real consent for a change in technique and enable us to free ourselves from confusion about what we are responsible for'.

Common to all four areas of work is the effort to understand the parents' experience of their particular child, and to explore with them how this is dependent not simply on their child's difficulties but on their unconscious interaction with the internal object worlds of their parents. This leads into discussion of the parents' own experiences as children. The technique involves close observation of the parental states of mind, and consideration of projective processes in the family and the ways in which vulnerabilities within the parents' personalities, and between them as a couple, become manifest and are enacted. The developing relationship with the parent therapist provides a way of understanding the underlying object relationships, and the parents' capacity to think about the infantile aspects of their child and of themselves. The way in which insights gained through transference and countertransference experiences are used varies depending on the nature of the work being undertaken.

What comes across so convincingly in Rustin's clinical vignettes is how psychoanalytic work with parents can lead to developmental growth in the parents as individuals, and as a couple, which has implications for them beyond becoming more effective parents to their troubled son or daughter. It is clear that work with parents undertaken in this way goes much further than what is often considered in clinics rather generically as 'support for parents'. This is psychoanalytic work in which the unconscious aspects of family life (including transgenerational inheritances) can be worked through, with the potential to develop more understanding and more satisfying family relationships. Rustin makes a strong case that those experienced in psychoanalytic work with children are very well placed to undertake this work.

Along with so many others, the editors of this book and the subsequent volume are fortunate to know, to have worked with, and to have been taught, supervised, and inspired by Margaret Rustin. Alongside her evident psychoanalytic capacities, many of Margaret's personal qualities – her generosity of heart, her determination of spirit, and her commitment to truth – permeate the papers presented here. We trust that the chapters which follow will provide readers with a vivid encounter with a distinctive clinician and thinker.

SECTION 1

THE SCOPE OF CHILD AND ADOLESCENT PSYCHOTHERAPY
Three case studies

1

FINDING OUT WHERE AND WHO ONE IS

The special complexity of migration for adolescents (2013)

Adolescence involves a major and disturbing shift in identity – both in how one is perceived and in how one experiences oneself. There is a normal and necessary re-working of one's place in the family, the move from the position of dependent child under the authority and protection of parental figures, towards a more independent status in which decisions can be taken about education and career direction, and about personal relationships. The adolescent can choose friendship groups and explore sexuality away from the reach of family. He or she is thus not only taking up a new position in the family but also placing him or herself in particular ways which shift and evolve through the adolescent years in the hugely important peer group and in relation to external social structures such as school, workplace and cultural context – and when things go wrong the health and social care and criminal justice systems.

What I hope to explore here is what happens when the pressures of this psycho-social transition of adolescence collide with the confusion, loss, disorientation and often traumatic elements characteristic of enforced migration. I shall discuss work with two adolescent boys both of whom had been thrown out of their known world by external circumstances. Their internal responses to this fact give a picture of how defensive psychic systems take shape, and how psychoanalytic psychotherapy may be able to free such adolescents from

DOI: 10.4324/9781003325543-3

the life-destroying aspects of their survival strategies. The two boys suffered different kinds of loss of home. The first was an asylum-seeking refugee from former Yugoslavia who had arrived in the UK together with his family after a traumatic flight from communal violence. The second was abandoned on the steps of social services by his mother at the age of eight and in long-term foster care since then. Both were seriously depressed when I first met them.

Working with such depressed young people is a great challenge for the therapist, especially when their access to effective adult support is very limited. In such cases, the therapist can feel assailed by a sense of loneliness, helplessness and alienation similar to the states of mind in her patient.

I do not think I had fully appreciated the ways in which my experience as a therapist for these boys would often leave me dependent on following my own thoughts and feelings in order to have anything to work with during the long silences within sessions and the frequently missed sessions which were to be so central a part of the therapeutic process. The fragmentation of experience, the isolation I felt and the intensity of my anxiety was I believe closely linked to the psychological impact on them of the distressing events which had preceded and also followed the loss of home.

In our major cities, there is a significant refugee population. There is limited experience to draw on in setting up services which will meet the needs of refugee families and children, and there is a troublingly hostile media-led growth of antagonism to refugees which has tended to be fanned rather than contained by the political leadership at the national level. This intensifies the mismatch between the level of need that it is only too easy to identify and the resources which can be made available: the fear of a backlash against any asylum provision makes it difficult for those commissioning and providing services to give much priority to a beleaguered minority, and in consequence a considerable proportion of the therapeutic interventions available are located in the voluntary sector, where humanitarian arguments have more impact. The Medical Foundation for Victims of Torture in London has, for example, been a major source of ideas about what sort of work is helpful for severely traumatized individuals. Nonetheless, there has been a modest growth in specialist provision for refugees, and I was asked to see the boy I shall now describe as part of the work of the Refugee team working in Child and Adolescent services at the Tavistock Clinic.

I think it will be helpful first to outline some concepts which are vital in providing a framework for understanding the refugee experience. As my focus is on the mental health needs of young refugees, the concepts I shall draw attention to are ones relevant to this aspect of their lives. It is nonetheless essential to keep in mind that a range of other perspectives are also needed to grasp the full picture – political, economic and social factors necessarily shape and influence the psychological domain.

It is with the idea of home and the meanings of loss of home that I shall start. A sense of home is to do with settledness, with having a place where one is unconditionally accepted. This fundamental place of safety can of course be lost for many reasons, but when large scale movements of refugees take place, we are dealing with whole communities who have lost their safe place, not just an aggregation of homeless individuals and families. The natural human response of sympathy is always stirred by images of displaced families – the television footage of thousands of Kosovan Albanians travelling helplessly undoubtedly played a part in bringing about European intervention in that conflict, for example. The violation of people's homes is felt as a moral outrage, even though war situations obscure this in some circumstances. Refugees' primary requirement is a place to be, sadly often temporary camps which can be all there is for many years, but whatever the place it will not be 'home' for them. It can over time become a new home, if recovery and the resumption of lives can take place, but there is a necessary lengthy period when loss of home will be a dominant preoccupation.

Home is a place of basic containment, the physical counterpart to the psychological function of the family. It provides a substratum of identity and its loss provokes anxieties of disorientation, collapse and loss of structure. A profound sense of insecurity or even of falling to pieces is a common experience. Esther Bick's metaphor of the unheld baby as being like a man in space without a spacesuit is a pertinent image to keep in mind. A profound sense of psychic insecurity can persist partly because the psychological pain of refugees is frequently defended against through processes of somatization. While the individual can appear rather frozen in mind, unable to think, we often get a vivid picture of bodies in pain. The mental distress is present in these disabling bodily symptoms, because the mind's capacity to contain emotional experience has become overwhelmed. As you will see, this is very evident in the case I shall be describing. Without the containment of the familiar home, the development of individuals, the regulation of interpersonal conflict within families and the established boundary between the privacy of the family (the area of intimacy) and the outside world all break down. This makes the non-homelike place of asylum one in which all the usual functions of the family are disrupted.

How does this description relate to the sometimes over-used concept of trauma? Trauma has important and specific meaning both in respect of physical wounds and in defining certain kinds of assault on the mind. However, it is not the case that all individuals are traumatized (except in the loose everyday use of the term) by becoming refugees. The balance of vulnerability and resilience within individuals and families plays a central role in determining whether the shocking experience of becoming refugees – of displacement from home – has a traumatic impact on the personality. When it does, a lengthy process of healing is required. The potential for self-healing will depend on the inner resources of individuals and communities, and of course be supported or impeded by the amount and type of help provided for them in their new place of abode. If the frightening insecurity of the original dislocation is replicated by the communal atmosphere and economic and political realities of their new setting, this undermines the potential process of recovery and stabilization. Being subject to the lengthy – even interminable – uncertainties of bureaucratic decision making about refugee status tends to keep people in a state of internal homelessness and create a kind of existence outside ordinary time. In fact the loss of the ordinary relationship to time is one of the recurrent difficulties for refugees waiting for an unpredictable period before they can begin living again in any ordinary way. This feature of their experience is reminiscent of children who have been accommodated following failure of care in their birth families. Such children have special difficulties in acquiring a working concept of time – temporal sequencing is confused, and the flow of time is disordered, sometimes for many years. It is as if their chaotic experience has cast them back into the timeless world of the small infant, and utterly disrupted the natural ordering of time which more fortunate children achieve. The mismatch between bureaucratic time and the intense anxieties of the stateless refugee is a similar phenomenon.

Particularly relevant for understanding the position of young refugees is the disruption of family organization which frequently follows flight from home. Role reversal, in which the children tend to look after their parents, is common. The children, through school, and because of their greater plasticity, learn a new language more easily. They become the interpreters. Living in two languages and two cultures can be a very complex experience. Eva Hoffman's marvellous book *Lost in Translation* (1989) is an exceptionally subtle account of a 13-year-old's experience of life in a Polish/Jewish community and the new world of North America and the English language. In more popular vein, Monica Ali's well-known novel *Brick Lane* (2003) offers a fictional representation of Bangladeshi life in London's East End in which the heroine lives in both her original homeland and her new home in her mind. The history of many migrations makes it evident that most people manage such transitions over time. Indeed the enriching of our and other national cultures has depended on just such movements of population. But within a family, the adults who can't manage the outside world lose status and authority. An asylum-seeking father has no right to work – but who is he without work? Mother with her usually more ready place in the lives of children in the community, at the shops, the school gate and so on, may find it a bit easier, but such differences in the position of man and wife may turn the marital relationship upside down. Certainly the enormously different attitudes to the role of women in modern and more traditional societies is one of the most difficult challenges facing many newly arrived families.

To look after young refugees more adequately than we have done, there are two very different groups to consider. Those arriving with families, or at least parts of families, are in a different position from the unaccompanied children who are a particularly vulnerable group. The latter have lost the ordinary representation of themselves as children who are being taken care of by adults, when the assumption is that the decisions belong to the grown-ups. Precocious responsibilities are thrust on children without family and yet it may be very hard for them to accept the alternatives provided by the authorities, which will feel so utterly unfamiliar.

Now I would like to introduce to you the 15-year-old boy whose story enabled me to grasp some of the specificities of the adolescent refugee experience.

Vorjat

Vorjat came to England as part of the Albanian flight from Kosovo. His family was, sadly, in a state of utter mental collapse. He was the only one of the four remaining family members who had been able to emerge into a partial integration into a life outside the home.

Vorjat's father was taken by Serb soldiers from his home as part of the intimidation of the local population. He was assaulted and kept prisoner for several weeks. Meanwhile his older brother, a student, was involved in university protests against what was taking place. He disappeared, and his disfigured dead body was discovered by his distraught mother subsequent to the violent suppression of student protest. The final horror was the arrival of Serb paramilitaries at the family home and the rape of mother in front of the two younger children, Vorjat and his older sister. When Father eventually returned, he rejected his wife as a consequence of the rape, a common response in this particular community. The family home was burnt to the ground before their eyes and they left their village with nothing.

I began once-weekly psychotherapy with Vorjat, following work by other colleagues in the multi-disciplinary team which revealed the following picture. Mother's mental health had totally collapsed. She was being cared for by a combination of medication and three days per week in a local psychiatric day centre. At a recent review meeting, it had emerged that she was barely able to dress herself or make a cup of tea. The impression was that the two children managed things at home, Soraya within the house, and Vorjat as the family's external representative. Father seemed despairing and terrified that his required weekly visits to the police station would one day result in his being detained and returned to Kosovo or imprisoned. Neither parent had been able to learn any English. They were thus dependent on interpreters or their son serving as interpreter in all contacts outside the home. Soraya was unable to leave the house and seemed crushed by the numerous blows the family had suffered. She was suffering from acute physical symptoms, with great difficulties in digesting any food. She was described as 'nothing but bones'.

Vorjat, however, believed in the idea that his family came here because they would get help, and he would get an education (both parents had been well-educated) and would then get a job.

He arrived on time for our first session after a long bus journey, a tidy, very clean, polite boy in school uniform. He seemed nervous and frequently wrung his hands as he described how everyone in the family is sick. He told me he goes to get mother's medicines for her – there would be no medicine if they are sent back to Kosovo. She would be dead if they had stayed there because there would have been no medical care for her. He knows no one there anymore. How would they live, he asked me, without a sense of rhetorical exaggeration. They have no house any more. There would be no money.

Later I asked him about school. Worriedly he said that sometimes he gets 'crazy'. People abuse him for being a refugee – 'Go home', they say. 'You're taking our houses', 'Why doesn't your father work?' and so on. Sometimes he can't bear this and gets into fights. Then he gets suspended, and his father gets angry with him and frightened that they will be in trouble. When I ask whether he can talk to anyone at school, he says 'no one knows about me'. There was one other refugee boy, but he has left. Vorjat doesn't know what has happened to him.

In this first meeting I spoke to him about his dislike of travel, picking up his vivid description of how sick he had felt on the bus. Noting how hard it was to get comfortable in my room, how tense he was feeling, I suggested it was difficult to cope with changes (a new room, me as a new therapist). But I mainly focused on the evident conflict between the part of himself that wants to try to make use of school – wants to go on to college and do well in exams – and wants to use the opportunity of coming to the Tavistock, and the contrary pull towards joining his family who he feels have all more or less given up. I suggested he was letting me know he was afraid he would decide it is not worth the difficult effort. I spoke about how lonely it makes him feel if he tries to make something of his life when the others can't manage this, and how worried he is about his rage and his problem in controlling this.

The following week was half-term and Vorjat got confused about which day of the week it was and rang to leave a message that he had got muddled and wouldn't be able to get to the clinic in time. That very week, the Home Secretary had announced his intention to allow families who had been living here as asylum seekers for more than three years to stay – I had been wondering how Vorjat would respond to this hopeful news.

He arrived on time for his next session. It took more than half the 50 minute session before he could tell me about this enormous change in the family circumstances. Before we got to that point, he spoke about feeling so sick on the bus journey. In Kosovo he never travelled on buses – school was next door to his house in the village. He walked everywhere. I linked his distress about the bus journey to the long journey to England and after a long silence he then told me about this – the journey was undertaken under a tarpaulin in the back of a lorry, and they only travelled at night. He would wonder whether the driver knew where they were. If they had tried to leave legally they would have been sent back and killed. Now he likes to imagine having a passport and being able to travel like other people – would he ever want to go back to his country? Or might he go one day somewhere else in Europe on holiday?

After more long pauses, he described to me the 'mock' exam at school yesterday. Everyone was terrified. Nobody knew it was going to happen. They were all taken into a big room with desks set out for the exam. His problem is spelling. He can speak and read quite well but spelling is difficult. Perhaps he might train as a mechanical engineer which wouldn't require him to be good at spelling – though he likes computers and IT.

In the last part of the session I hear of his phoning the solicitor and of the social worker's visit to the family. Three times he tells me that he won't be sure of the news until they get the letter. I am able to explore with him the profundity of his distrust of what sounds like good news. I privately think to myself that his failing to come to the second appointment may well have been an enactment of his doubts about my reliability – was he testing out whether I meant it that he would have a weekly session with me? To my surprise, as he left he said 'see you next week, if you haven't forgotten me' which exactly expresses this point. The letter he awaits will come from authorities who he fears may have forgotten his existence – he feels he has become a non-person, during this long wait. However, by contrast he speaks of the social worker who arranged re-housing for the family with great appreciation. I realize that the task for me as therapist is to bring together these two sides of his way of seeing the world, to help him to modify his paranoid suspicion and despair by linking it with contrasting good experience which he recognizes as benign. His personal optimism will then have more of a chance. At this moment I have a sense of what our work will be about, and am quite hopeful about it.

If I try to capture the essence of these first contacts, it is to do with the balance of hope and hopelessness. The sad and lonely feeling expressed by his rather limp, slightly placatory demeanour (as if not to offend at all costs), by his choice of the chair in my room closest to the door – farthest from me, barely making a claim on my time and attention, and also ready to make a quick getaway – by the stillness of his body and low inexpressive tone of his voice, all these were offset and lightened by the smile that occasionally lit up his face.

What was particularly difficult to comprehend was the meaning he attached to evidence of there being something worth hoping for, something that could change for the better. I began to grasp that one aspect of this was that ordinary impulses to fight for survival, to assert oneself, are inhibited for a variety of reasons. When good news arrives, it seems to offer an opportunity for a part of himself that has gone into a kind of hibernation to reappear. But that is a very dangerous moment. What enabled me to get hold of this problem was a puzzling set of conversations further exploring the misery of the bus journey to the clinic. The experience of feeling sick seemed an inescapable part of getting to his session. The slowness and unreliability of the bus services was a regular source of persecution. I began to think about the literal facts of his journey and to find myself dying to tell him that he could come by underground much more quickly. So powerful was the desire to take him out of the place of persecution (being stuck on the bus) that my comments to him about this feeling undoubtedly had a leading question aspect to them – had he considered other ways of getting here? Did he feel sick on trains in the same sort of way? The pressure to act out and offer specific help became irresistible, at one point. Our discussion got very concrete and I found myself (to my alarm) explaining that the Jubilee line underground was not the only one close to the clinic – the Northern line, more accessible from his home, which stopped at Belsize Park would be an alternative. At the time Vorjat looked rather eager about this idea and indeed asked me to write down the name of the station for him, which I decided to do, but I was feeling painfully uneasy about what was happening between us, aware that my over-interest in a less troubling journey for him probably felt to him like evidence of my not being able to tolerate the unending misery he was telling me about. I also felt worried that I was taking over an ego function quite inappropriately, although I excused myself by reflecting on the absence of appropriate external support for him. His world did not seem to contain parents who could help with ordinary things like travel arrangements, and my acting-out was a response to this. To make me even more anxious about what I had done, I was faced the following week with his absence – I received a message to say that he had to visit his sister in hospital. Whatever the real external aspects of this (and I do not want to underestimate the importance of her serious symptoms of sleeplessness, weight loss and continuous vomiting) I felt clear that I had let down my patient in my failure to hold on to his hopelessness. Instead of bringing the ill aspect of himself to the clinic for my attention, he had shifted into an identification with me, becoming the one who has to look after someone else. As he has his session on a school morning, his hospital visit also meant he was not going to school, so there was a double loss – no therapist and no teachers for him. Instead he was having to be the carer for his family, to take on the missing parental functions.

A new aspect emerged when he told me for the first time of the details of what had happened in Kosovo before they left. He knew I had a broad sense of this from the clinic file and my colleagues, but it seemed very important that he himself put words to these grim events. What struck me particularly was his picture of his older brother, the student killed in the police repression of student protest. There was a palpable sense of the younger boy's admiration of his big brother, the clever law student, the one willing to stand up for people's rights. At the same time, the evidence seemed to be that resistance to oppression and assertion of oneself was deadly dangerous. Being willing to fight was mixed up, for Vorjat, with a dread of catastrophe. He spoke again of his anxiety about 'losing it' when he feels provoked by other boys at school, and described a fight when he felt blind with rage and had to be pulled off another boy whom he was pummelling to a ferocious degree. The difficulty of being in touch with his aggression in any controllable way was manifest, and the problem for me was how to link up his ever-grateful conscious attitude to me, the only feeling of which he was aware, with other very different feelings pushed to one side.

As we approached the first holiday break, I felt most anxious about how any link would be maintained. He came neither to the two last pre-Xmas sessions, nor to the first of the New Year. As usual I wrote to him acknowledging each absence and reminding him that I would hope to see him the following week. I found myself puzzling over these apparently brief and simple letters, spending a long time to find the phrase that felt right – not too much or too little, was my aim.

When he returned in January, he was in very low spirits. I gradually clarified that he thought I would be fed up by his many absences and would cut the frequency of his sessions in consequence. There was an atmosphere of great difficulty about remembering anything and much depression about whether it was worth hoping for anything. In particular, the family had still not heard from the Home Office. Vorjat also began, for the first time, to talk of having to give up his hopes of going to college after he finished his GCSEs. He will have to get a job to support his family for if they get passports and legal status, they will lose benefits. No one else in the family can work, so it will depend on him. When he did remember why he had not been able to come last week, he explained he had had to take his father to hospital for an appointment for bladder investigation.

The following week brought a surge of hope with the arrival of the Home Office letter. 'I got here' he said happily, as he sat down at the beginning of the session, and he had arrived on time. For the very first time, I had a picture of some ordinary life in the family – 'My father woke me at 7.30. The letter had arrived and he wanted me to read it. I had forgotten to put on my alarm clock for coming here, and I was asleep. I read it to him three times. We have to go the solicitor to fill in the forms'. Later in the session he told me about a terribly bad stomach pain he has and his intention to go to the GP. At the time, I noted to myself that for once he seemed to be the one who might receive care (from me and from his GP) but I think it is also very relevant to note the probable somatization of the anxiety evoked by hope, and the unbearably painful quality of taking in something which might lead to growth and change.

In succeeding weeks, there were continuing references to sources of support for hopeful feelings – a helpful solicitor who replaced the one who seemed to have forgotten them and gone off on maternity leave, stories of two teachers at school who had given him encouraging feedback in contrast to the usual idea that there is no one to understand. But the threat to this possible improvement in his prospects, external and internal, remained. Many sessions were cancelled (although one cancellation when Vorjat's sister rang me up to say that he was ill in bed made me feel less worried, since she seemed to be able to help to look after him by phoning me) and I struggled to work out what I felt I was being left with.

Thinking about the meaning of absence by a patient is always hard. When Vorjat did not come, I believe he was giving me some psychic work to do on his behalf. His absence might be one that left me in the dark (no message, or only one that arrives after the time of his session); perhaps in that state of not-knowing I am put in touch with the sort of experience he has had in recent years of not knowing what is going to happen to him and his family in the legal process. More darkly, it has the resonance of his family's terrifying experience when both father and then brother disappeared and left a household with no idea of where they were or whether they would return. The dread I am aware of on the mornings of his session is intense. I long for him to get here safely but have a gnawing anxiety that he won't. This is not like the ordinary experience of waiting for an adolescent patient. Perhaps my countertransference reaction is a response both to Vorjat's own fears of possible loss and anxious emptiness but also to the state of his internal mother, a mother whose mind has been blown to bits by an excess of traumatic losses. I feel myself to be a therapist who may be losing contact with her patient in a life-threatening way.

Another thread in my thoughts is the issue of guilt and responsibility. I have touched on this already in discussing what I felt to be my mistake when we were talking about how he could manage the journey. More distressing to me was the question about whether a three week absence had been provoked by a change to the time of his session that I had had to make. At the time, it was not evident that this disruption of routine might be risky. In fact rather otherwise, since in negotiating the alternative time we arranged, Vorjat was actually able to indicate that my first proposal was not good for him – in other words, to express a preference rather than to be compliantly accepting. So he came to the changed appointment with apparent equanimity. However, I had to ask myself the question as to whether his subsequent absence was related to unconscious anger which could only be expressed in this passive way. What alerted me to the likelihood of such hostility and protest being a part of what was going on was the discomfort I have felt plagued by in relation to my team colleagues. I found myself exceptionally irritated by the mistakes made by the team secretary in typing letters (my title, or the day of the week being confused and necessitating re-typing) but even worse by a conviction that it was when other meetings are arranged in which my colleagues were in reality attempting to support the family as a whole – the link-up with Vorjat's mother's day hospital, for example – that he did not come to see me. I think there may have been something in my idea that two clinic-related appointments in one week couldn't be managed and that it was his therapy session that got sacrificed as he settled himself into the role of the interpreter or carer for his parents and lost contact with his own needs. But what intrigued me was my irrational anger with my colleagues who of course were playing their part in looking after this distressed family but appeared to me as competitors for the opportunity to do any effective work. I felt helpless, left waiting for someone who does not arrive, frustrated and also jealous that others can be effective while I couldn't. This rather unusual countertransference points to the extent of Vorjat's difficulties in expressing negative feelings of any kind towards me.

The empty session's capacity to stir dread is something to do with the fear that something has died. The penumbra of endless mourning is also very much suggested by the grey and black clothes Vorjat wears (partly, but not wholly determined by school uniform) and his very pale skin, giving the impression of skin not much exposed to the light.

Occasionally I got a glimpse of his own feeling of unsureness about the ongoingness of life. The sense of being forgotten and becoming a non-person in the eyes of powerful authorities was one example of this threat to existence. A second example concerned his school. Vorjat attended a school subject to 'special measures' (a most unhelpful external echo of his internal insecurity) and he told me that he had learnt that his school was to close. He went on to imagine a future in which he and other ex-pupils would be telling people where they went to school and no one would be able to understand because the school would have vanished. He was able to explain that he thought the building would have been pulled down and that there would be simply no evidence that the school he went to ever existed. Now we could hear and track the resonance of the lost home and destroyed village in Kosovo, but I was also struck by the picture of his sharing this situation with others who would also have lost their school. The absoluteness of his loneliness seemed to me modified at this moment.

One of the other ideas I kept in mind in the silent spaces within sessions – the long pauses in which I was left wondering if what I had said has struck any chord or not – is the matter of Vorjat's living in two languages. At home, English is a foreign language. At school, he learnt pretty good English and conversationally there was no problem – he seemed linguistically like any London schoolboy. However, the silences in our conversations might represent some complex process of inner translation and processing. Some colleagues using interpreters have noted the helpful function of the space created by the time required for the interpreter to speak, and suggested that this slowing down of the process contributes to modulating the level of pain that the exploration of traumatic experience entails.

Now I want to compare this clinical situation with one in which I came to see my patient as something like a refugee in his own country.

Wayne

Wayne was an Afro-Caribbean boy of 14 living in foster care and attending a school for children with moderate learning difficulties when I first met him. He had been brought up by his mother until he was eight years old, and abandoned to the care of social services at that point. I learnt about Wayne's picture of this only after more than a year of therapy. He believed that she had had some trouble and had left him at the social services office temporarily and then been unable to find her way back to collect him. He felt she was still looking for him but had got lost, and that all kinds of accidents had prevented them ever linking up again – the office had moved, she had arrived after it closed for the day, a message had got mislaid and so on. He gave the impression of a life spent waiting patiently. In the meantime, he had some contact with his father, grandfather and a large collection of brothers and uncles and aunts – children of his father by other women were all described as his brothers. One in particular, a boy of four or five, who lived with his young mother seemed especially important, and when this couple left to live in Barbados, Wayne was palpably bereft.

He had been referred for therapy because of his troubling level of depression. He was a profoundly sad boy, almost emotionally inert in his failure to reveal any feelings about anything. It seemed likely that his limited intellectual functioning was closely linked to the depths of his depression. His whole vital system seemed to have been closed down to produce a situation where he survived, but only just. He walked slowly and wearily, his body was limp in tone, his face expressionless, and he hardly spoke. His silence had led to the provision of speech therapy at his special school but seemed in fact to be the near-autism of a child whose mind had dropped to a very low level of activity. He was capable of almost complete lifeless inertia – sitting as if in a timeless world without movement or sound for extended periods.

When I met him, the trauma of abandonment, which I came to see as totally fundamental to his state, had unfortunately been repeated in the therapeutic setting due to the unexpectedly premature ending of work by a previous therapist. To her amazement, after long months of very, very little sign of life, in the final session Wayne made an eloquent plea for help. Though there were few words, powerful projective identification seized hold of her and this led to a conviction that a new therapist must be found. The waiting-list pressure imposed a delay of many months, but I was then able to pick up the case.

Earlier in this chapter, I have been exploring the question of what happens when trauma enters the consulting room very concretely. In Wayne's case the problem was the degree of his passivity. This had the impact on me of evoking either a near deadly drift into an empty-minded state, in which all sense of life ebbed away, or of provoking irritability, and pressures in the countertransference to poke and prod and demand a response. This was manifestly counterproductive since I could observe that any enlivened or magnified communication from me caused him to shrink further down inside himself. It was extremely hard to maintain a level of interest and a sense of hopefulness that there could be some point in the sessions. Trying to understand this state as one communicated non-verbally by my patient, within which I was almost engulfed, did not seem to lead to my being able to formulate anything meaningful to him. Speaking about feelings of any sort seemed to be felt as a threat, but the presentation was more as if this sort of talking was an utterly foreign language, however simply I couched my interpretations.

The intense loneliness I experienced was added to by the weak sense of life around Wayne. His social worker had arranged for him to be brought by an escort to the clinic. I had met his foster-mother once before beginning work. She was a grandmotherly figure with grown-up children and grandchildren, and prepared to go along with what the authorities suggested, but there seemed little evidence of life between her and Wayne. My experience in therapy soon suggested to me some of the reasons for her retreat into a position of limited involvement. Wayne's social worker left soon after I started work. My phone calls and letters to social services fell into a bottomless pit of non-response, and when he stopped being brought to his sessions just before the first holiday break, I had no one to link with. Foster-mother had gone to Jamaica for a protracted visit, there was no social worker, and Wayne did not respond to my letters. The sense of hopeless re-enactment which could not be resisted was colossal. It was the very session after the one when I spoke to him about my Christmas holiday that he failed to arrive. I was sure he felt I was leaving him – but then so were all the significant figures with potential parental responsibility in the external world.

Coming to life again

For about a term, I struggled between enraged attempts to achieve a response from social services or the foster-family and a powerful sense of futility and despair which pressed me towards giving up. The other children on the waiting list, the fact that the time I had given him was in reality a difficult one for me to protect from other demands and the memory of the painful effort I had to make in sessions to stay alive to what was going on in the room all conspired to create a drift towards giving up. Somehow I did not, and kept open his session time. To my astonishment, one day I got a phone call from the foster-mother's daughter, who was looking after the household while her mother was away. She told me she was worried about Wayne. She knew he needed to come to the clinic so that he could be helped to express himself. She promised to bring him next week. Though very late, they did arrive – a lively young woman, her two children (18 months and three) bursting with energy, and Wayne as large and limp as ever. Because there were so few minutes left and it was many months since we had met, I decided to use the time to talk to Wayne and his foster-sister together about trying to get the therapy re-established.

In the months that followed, there was never quite such a close shave with the death of the therapy, though very numerous smaller-scale repetitions. But I want to concentrate on describing an aspect of how I came to try to work. I saw that I had to investigate the imbalance between my sense of desperate effort to make contact and his mute retreatism. I struggled to slow down my words, to simplify sentences, to leave great amounts of time for a possible response from him and to use any fragment of verbal communication from Wayne as a building block. We started to have conversations about how he couldn't think – his experiences of losing his thoughts, which at times we could see happening in sessions, and which I could try and link to the emotional significance of the lost thought. Tiny moments of spontaneous activity occurred, hoarded anxiously by me as providing evidence of potential growth in Wayne's impoverished mind.

Eventually a new social worker appeared on the scene and played a helpful role in supporting the idea that Wayne might make the journey to the clinic on his own. He was now 16, and going to college. Despite many ups and downs, this shift was made, and it led to Wayne being able to talk to me about what happened to him on his way to the clinic. He usually came quite late, and I talked through with him what had gone on. He would explain about setting off from college (probably late already) and getting muddled about trains and stations then distracted by shops he passed and so on. One week soon after this he was ill and to my excitement he rang up the clinic and spoke to say he would not be able to come. He explained that he thought I would wonder where he was and be worried and that he wanted me to know what had happened. Another week, when, exceptionally, he arrived on time, I saw him glance at the clock in the corridor as he walked to my room. This, I felt, was a reproach to me as I had kept him waiting in the waiting room for two minutes, due to an urgent phone call. He almost acknowledged this when I referred to it.

There was one session which highlighted for me a significant factor in his emergence from his traumatized half-life and his greater access to his own mental life. He was telling me about his journey to the clinic, including almost smiling as he described going into a stationery shop to buy stuff he needed for college and his awareness that this would make him late. He seemed in touch with the aggressive aspect of choosing to keep me waiting and linked this to the 'forgetting' of what his foster-mother asks him to do at home – he gets up to respond but cannot remember what it is so then cannot do it. We talked at length about what had happened next in the station. He needed to get a Jubilee line train, but he was interested in the Metropolitan line going to Uxbridge (the opposite direction).

He was wondering where the trains were coming from, where they were going to (almost like a little boy train spotter). He was aware that, as he watched them, he was missing Jubilee line trains. The two sets of railway tracks intrigued him.

I could see the process of what he had always experienced as forgetting (something like dropping into black holes in his mind) becoming an active turning away. I felt I could describe to him his identification with a figure going-off-in-the-opposite-direction – like Mrs Rustin at the end of a session, like mother a long time ago – who leaves the Wayne who wants to get here and be with me stranded and deprived of most of his session. Better to be the forgetter, than the forgotten one.

But the most interesting thing is that the two tracks of thinking, like the two sets of railway lines, are simultaneously available to Wayne's inner vision. The sense of absolute loss of mindfulness has been replaced momentarily by a vision of choice and direction, and of awareness of the consequence of going one way or the other.

I think the rage, fear, hatred and consequent guilt this boy might have experienced in relation to his abandonment was so terrible that there was a massive closing down of his mind. In treatment, I was brought very close to re-enactment of the abandonment many times, in small ways within and between sessions and in gross ways in terms of the repeated efforts I had to make to sustain the therapy and the temptation to give up. The powerful feelings I refer to were mostly evoked in me – rage with social services' inadequacies, for example, guilt about the near repetitions that kept happening and hatred of the passivity I witnessed which evoked my aggression. I was powerfully reminded at times of the dynamic of relationships between enslaved peoples and their all-powerful masters. All sense of potency often seemed to lie with me, and none with Wayne. The sort of boredom and emptiness one faces in sessions with silent passive patients like this is a chilling challenge to one's equanimity. Too little anger about the waste of a life will lead to a deadly collusion, an enacted abandonment of the live child, too free an expression of it to frozen terror in the patient, whose belief is that the life in him was responsible for all he had lost – mother couldn't cope with him, he was too much for her; the only hope of holding on to someone is to be an inoffensive mouse.

These two boys, both at the time of treatment at an age where ordinarily adolescent passions, excitement and discomfort might be expected, faced me instead with a state of depressed inertia which I would describe as a psychic failure to thrive. The perpetual threat of the death of the therapy was the core clinical issue and the mode by which their earlier traumatic losses and their psychic consequences could be approached. The devastating way in which dreadful external events had penetrated and damaged their minds and the ongoing failings and cruelties of the systems on which they were dependent made for many technical difficulties in the therapy – the differentiation between internal and external reality was not easy to make, and the pressure on the therapist to focus too much attention and feeling on external problems was continuous. Getting the balance wrong would only add an additional layer of failure to provide what was required.

I think it will be evident how profoundly disturbing it was to be in touch with the unbearable aspects of these two lives, but to help these boys to bear things in a realistically hopeful spirit was my task. I believe what helped me was the effort to describe – to find words for my thoughts and observations, the majority of which were private to myself, part of an internal conversation. The concept of the unbearable brings to mind Bion's phrase 'nameless dread'. If it can be named, it is defused of some of its power and can then be further investigated, become an object of thought. Without this process of thinkability, such young people are vulnerable to dangerous degrees of violent emotion which can either be turned inwardly against the self (as is so evident in Wayne's case), or may erupt in violent enactment as sometimes happened with Vorjat. I was disturbed to learn that two of the would-be bombers in London on July 21st 2005 were refugees from Eritrea and Somalia, who had arrived in Britain as young adolescents fleeing from horrific civil wars. The globalization of all our lives makes it urgent that we think hard about the risks facing young people burdened by unbearable experiences in communities where the adults are often totally unable to provide containment. The combination of inter-generational breakdown in families and international failures of responsibility leaves a dangerous void. Psychoanalytic thinking can, however, enable us to begin to understand the internal processes which can traumatic loss into something so terrible that it can only lead to a form of repetition compulsion in which both self and other will be trapped in torment and devastation.

2

IDENTITY THEMES IN PSYCHOTHERAPY WITH AN ADOPTED MIXED RACE ADOLESCENT (1989)

Freud's great paper "Mourning and Melancholia" (1917 [1915]) is the well-known starting point for the psychoanalytic theory of internal objects. His central insight was to link the state of melancholia or pathological mourning with the individual's relationship to the lost object. Instead of being able to accept the reality of the loss of the dead person, to experience grief, to mourn, and to re-engage with the world and make new relationships, the melancholic individual remains pre-occupied with what is lost (usually another person, but in some cases an idea or belief system, or a conception of self) and lives a life overshadowed by this loss. In Freud's much quoted and poetic phrase: "The shadow of the object [falls] upon the ego". Freud's theory, developed more fully by Abraham and later Klein, suggested that the ambivalent relationship to the lost object was the core difficulty, and that the unconscious angry reproaches of the mourner held him prisoner. Abraham linked these ideas to the vicissitudes of the early mother-child relationship and Klein's remarkable papers on mourning (1935, 1940, 1945) expanded our understanding of the self's relationship to internal figures to delineate a detailed picture of the internal world. She described a world within the child's mind peopled by maternal, paternal and sibling figures formed through internalisation of family relationships as experienced by the child and shaped by unconscious phantasy.

DOI: 10.4324/9781003325543-4

This is the fundamental theoretical background to much of psychoanalytic child psychotherapy, elaborated by many later writers. This paper draws particular attention to the importance of the relationship between the internal parents – what sort of a couple they are felt to be. This theme was written about by Harris and Meltzer (1976) in an original way and more recently explored by Britton (1989), who has been interested in the links between the capacity for thought and the oedipal constellation. A triangle in which mother and father are perceived to be together by the observing child and to have independent links to the child is, he argues, the basis for mental health.

This theory has proved particularly helpful in understanding the states of mind we encounter in the many neglected, deprived and maltreated children now seen by child psychotherapists. To add to the complexity, these children often have multiple parental figures due to family breakdown, and their internal world reflects this confusion.

The adolescent whose treatment I want to describe had a chaotic early life. He lived in a world of unpredictable care, neglect and violence, but he was certainly also a child loved by his mother in her own way. He was therefore not a child without a conception of being wanted and a child with a sense of himself as worthy of love and capable of loving. However, at the time of referral by his social worker and adoptive parents, what was evident was the inner constellation that psychotherapists had begun to understand in children removed from inadequate parental care who could not then make use of the good substitute care in their new family. These were the children who suffered from the "double deprivation" identified by Gianna Henry in her classic paper (1974). The extended deprivation and destructiveness of their earlier life circumstance was added to by an inner situation in which, for various reasons, the child was so profoundly identified with the damaging original parental objects that there was a huge barrier to the development of new relationships which could provide for the necessary dependent needs of the child. These children seemed stuck in the past in their inner selves in a way that walled them off from the potential benefit of their new circumstances. Their states of mind tended to undermine the hopefulness and strength of the new parental figures within their substitute families and thus to bring about a repetition of the earlier damage. In these dangerous situations, psychotherapeutic intervention can sometimes serve to first contain and ultimately transform through slow processes of development the inner parental figures of the child's internal world.

Max was born to a young single white mother in Holland. His father was said to be a black sailor who disappeared before he was born by which time Mother was living with another boyfriend. This relationship also broke up, and Max's own memories are of two other men with whom Mother lived before he was taken into care aged four. Mother was a drug addict, living a tenuous existence. She became addicted to heroin as well as using many other drugs, and was often unable to take care of herself or Max. He has memories of being in hospital at about two and a half for malnutrition, and of resisting Mother's attempts to dress him in wet clothes picked up on the streets. When Max was approaching four, he and his mother were sent to stay overnight with a family who had offered help to an agency trying to rehabilitate homeless drug addicts. This family became much involved with Max and his mother, initially in trying to help and support them as a pair, and subsequently offering to become the adoptive parents for the boy, when they became convinced that his mother's dilapidated life was unlikely to be open to change, and that it was having very damaging effects on Max. This arrangement was confirmed by the courts, and Max has remained the foster child of this family since then.

The family which took him in was composed of white middle-class business and professional parents, and their three natural children, two boys older than Max, and a girl a little younger. Soon after the court decision, Father was asked to move to London for a while by his firm. The Tavistock was contacted by a social work agency, with a request for treatment for Max. An assessment of Max (now aged seven) and the family led to a decision to offer him intensive psychotherapy, and regular work was also offered to the parents.

He began treatment with one of my colleagues when he was seven and a half. He suffered from asthma and frequent illnesses, terrifying nightmares, and many anxieties about school, but pre-eminent was his repeated wish to go and live with his mother. He could not understand or accept the impossibility of this; his parents were tormented by the implicit rejection of their loving efforts as he repeatedly asked, "Why can't I live with my mother?" His therapist found him a very available little boy, full of imagination and eager to share his anxieties, but she was faced, as was his family, with the debilitating effects of his idealisation of his mother. In his mind, he had a protective relationship to Mother: in phantasy he was the rich prince who would rescue an abandoned or imprisoned princess; he blamed his adoptive family for separating him from his mother. There seemed to be several factors underpinning this idealisation: if Max gave it up, he would have to face the pain of his partial abandonment when he was four, and acknowledge the grim picture of his mother that went with this knowledge. Idealisation had protected him from the primitive anxieties of being devoured and torn to pieces which were documented in horror stories of cosmic proportions in his play and in his frightening dreams. Most problematically, the clinging to this idealisation, in which so much of himself was invested, protected him from the risks of genuine dependency on his new family or his therapist. Added to this were the seductive delights of a belief in a reunification with Mother on the basis of his role as the prince-rescuer which enabled him to evade all the oedipal issues that faced him in his new family, and the pains of sibling rivalry, which for him were almost unbearable. For he was, and remained throughout childhood, very upset about the differential status of natural and adopted children, and he could not of course even pretend he was one of the family's children in an ordinary way because of his dark skin. The tortured sense of himself as an outsider seems to have driven him back to his idyllic phantasies of reunion with Mother.

The work in his first period of therapy enabled him gradually to face some facts about his mother's life. On his visits to her (this was an open adoption, with continuing contact with Mother and her wider family) he could see that she lived in a terrible mess, was always ill, could not sleep, and took many pills. But this acknowledgement of reality faced him with his own rage at her failure to take care of him, and he became terrified of the volcanic anger which might erupt. A desire to take care of her was also powerfully evoked. He was unable to hold on to his anger and struggled to protect his image of Mother and locate blame elsewhere: "She didn't know she was giving me bad things", "someone gave her the pills", he would say. A particularly horrific visit culminated in Mother following him to the airport, clinging to him physically so that he missed the plane.

The struggle in therapy to help Max reintegrate his repeatedly denied understanding of his mother's problems was terribly painful for both child and therapist. The therapist felt she was taking away from him what he loved most (namely the idealised image of Mother) and he felt she was forcing him to bear unbearable feelings. Also important, and this is central to the problems that he faced later, was his image of his father who had disappeared before his birth. Max's picture of this was that his father had lost him and his mother, and was still searching for them. This image of a forlorn and desperate wandering father was counterpointed by images of violent, drugged, and murderous male figures. A visit to Madame Tussaud's (the London waxwork museum) gave him dreadful nightmares and he explained that he always lay very still in bed so that if murderers came into his room they would not realise he was there.

Max's sense of difference, alienation, and isolation within his family was something he could talk about in a way that was quite unusual for a boy of his age, and his formulations were poignant. For example, he said: "I don't go in this family. I knew before I came to the Tavistock that I don't go in this family". He was aware of the traumatic effects of his separation from his mother. Of himself, he could say, "Some people stop growing when they are three or four and they don't look right", and he contrasted himself with other children: "Other children say 'I'm going to do this with my Mummy' or 'I'm going to do this with my Daddy' but I can never say that".

Max's therapy, which lasted four years, enabled him to turn more towards his new family, and when it ended he seemed to be doing quite well in his outside life. However, there remained a thought in his therapist's mind that in later adolescence he might need further help. The renegotiation of a child's sense of self under the impact of different developmental stages, especially in the face of the great changes of adolescence is, I think, closely linked to the nature and evolution of the parental couple in the mind. As adolescents experience the pressure of sexual desires, their picture of the intercourse of their parents is fundamental to the relationships they are able to embark on.

My assessment of Max

There were periodic review meetings with his therapist over the years when Max sometimes seemed to be asking for more, but this never came to anything until just before his 16th birthday. I was then asked to meet him to explore his request for further help. When he came to see me I encountered a tall, well-built young man with light brown skin and curly Afro hair, giving an impression of a gentle giant. He was distant and uneasy. He talked readily, but the interview was punctuated by his disagreeing very politely with almost any comment I offered, while at the same time conveying a needy feeling and making me feel under enormous pressure to get things right, which I manifestly could not do. The essence of the situation was that he wanted me to know that he needed help, for he told me about quite a number of areas of difficulty in his current life, but also that he could not accept it. The one thing I did that seemed to be right was to describe this impasse and to respond to it by accepting his adolescent need to work things out for himself and by proposing that we arrange to meet six months hence to see how he was getting on in this task. This he seemed pleased with, wanting me to take the responsibility of making that appointment. When we did meet again, a very similar sequence ensued: the range of troubles had changed somewhat, but the paradoxical message was the same. I again offered a meeting six months hence which he accepted. By this time I had a firm feeling that I would have a patient eventually, but that it was extremely important to wait, holding this very loose link, until he himself was ready to come closer. One could say that I needed to tolerate rejection while still being aware of his underlying need and provide a clinical response which took both into account.

In the third session the pattern shifted and we had a different sort of conversation. Max had come to say quite plainly that he was stuck. He had not in fact, he said, made any progress in working out the various problems he had and had decided that he now urgently wanted to get some help with this. There was a palpable sense of anxiety about time passing and of waste. He was now 17. He had done poorly in his exams – he is a bright boy, but had consistently underachieved at school. He felt badly about this, about his poor prospects in comparison with his siblings, his lack of friends, his unproductive conflicts with his mother, his awareness that he should be moving towards independence, and his humiliating sense of immobility. I said that I could offer him a weekly session, and we discussed whether he felt that this would be enough – in his previous period of therapy he had attended four times a week. I added that if this did prove a real difficulty, at a later stage I might be able to increase sessions. If he preferred,

I offered to find a colleague who could give him more than one weekly session now. He accepted the vacancy with me. I also told him that I thought he might like to use the couch when we began, to make the transition from these exploratory meetings with me to a commitment to ongoing therapy, and in recognition of the difference there would be in the work we would do now and the earlier work as a child with his previous therapist. I had in mind the acute discomfort in being looked at which I had noticed in making this suggestion to him.

So we began work. I must now fill in some important events in his life in the intervening years. When he was twelve his mother died from a complex form of hepatitis. Max told me that his mother's liver had been completely destroyed by her drug abuse. At about the same time, his adoptive parents split up. His father returned to their home country, while Mother remained in London with the children. Both parents later acquired new stable partners.

In his first few sessions, he gradually introduced me to his world. Nearest the surface was his adolescent conflict with his mother. There were bitter arguments about smoking; about how often he should go out in the evening and what time he needed to return. At one level these sounded absolutely typical of any teenage rebel. However, it was not quite like that – the stakes were very high, because Max felt that the implicit threat was always that he would be chucked out of the house forever. His judgement about this was probably distorted by his own powerful sense that he should be preparing to leave. This he also brought directly to me at the outset: he explained that he would be in London for a further two years. After that he intended to return to Holland. I thought he was trying to circumscribe the amount of attachment that he might come to feel towards me, to structure it carefully from the beginning so that he would be able to leave. There was certainly some problem on his mother's side too; she was perhaps terrified of his smoking because she felt it as the first step towards drugs and addiction. Despite all these arguments at home there was warmth between them; Max was aware of not wanting to hurt her and of wanting to leave home in a good way. Much more difficult were his relations with the rest of the family. He felt very much belittled by his siblings, mocked for his ideas, particularly his political convictions, not taken seriously, not treated as an equal. "Conversations stop when I come in", he said. He saw himself as an uncouth child, who does not know how to speak properly, what clothes to wear or how to eat, still at some level the poor child picked up off the streets.

Identity themes

In the first few months of our work, Max revealed several important identity conflicts and confusions. The old theme of whether he was one of the proper children, a family child, with equal rights and prospects, was an open wound. Many sessions dealt with his feelings of exclusion and his tendency to a paranoid interpretation of the ordinary ups and downs of family life. We were able to explore a long-standing failure to stand up for himself, due to his extreme anxiety about rejection, which always made him afraid of expressing any anger. This had made him collusive with abusive treatment from his siblings, a self-destructive collusion which now disgusted him. A related difficulty was his relatively poor academic performance. Teachers were consistently confident that he could do much better work, while Max oscillated between an arrogant intellectual superiority, much despair at his actual achievements, and huge problems in getting down to work. He was now studying for the International Baccalaureate, and in fact he did well (and a good deal better than his adoptive brothers) in his final exams, and this made a huge difference to his sense of status in the family.

A second source of anxiety was his confusion about his sexuality. His brothers teased him that he must be homosexual since he had no girlfriend, and he was tormented about this. He tried to prove his 'normality' by acquiring girl friends that he could show off. He then either kept them at a great distance, where they could be perceived as people in their own right but the relationship could not get off the ground, or he plunged into a sexual relationship which seemed to lack any warmth or personal feeling at all, leaving him as lonely as ever. Gradually he began to talk to me about his attraction to boys. He could not sort out whether he wanted a friendship or a sexual attachment, or how these two things could be linked, but as he became less frightened of finding out, he gathered courage to explore what might happen.

Other concerns included his political affiliations and his family's mockery and disapproval of these. He had come to define himself as a socialist, and joined a Trotskyist sect, which was eager to channel his energies in activity. He experienced a sense of belonging to "the party", as he called it, but while he enjoyed the way this affiliation structured his rows at home and the sense of moral superiority it engendered, he was upset both by the evidence of his own lack of consistent effort and by his recurrent awareness that his loneliness seemed little assuaged by all this activity. There was also the issue of where he belonged geographically, in London or Holland, and with which family; with his adoptive mother and siblings, or with his adoptive father and stepmother, or with the relatives of his natural mother with whom relationships had been maintained? He spent time in all these settings and was very muddled about the transitions from one to the other, which he made me experience vividly, as all his plans for visits to Holland were made at extremely short notice and thus his absences from therapy could never be thought about beforehand. It was however notable that he was totally unable to stay until the end of a term with me or to return for a first session after a holiday break, and the travelling to and fro thus became linked with the sense of homelessness in relation to me that was evoked by any discontinuities in the therapy. Messages to me about his absences always came after the event, if at all, and it seemed that for years the worry and uncertainty about broken links had to be registered in my mind and were out of Max's reach.

It will have been noted that I have not yet referred to feelings about racial identity, and this is because for a very long time this was not something with which he was consciously concerned. It did however preoccupy me considerably, and this was because although he did not talk about it at all or respond in words to anything I said on this theme for the first couple of years of therapy, his behaviour made it clear how crucial it was. For example, he got involved with his political group in fly-posting details of meetings and demonstrations in the Notting Hill area (a part of London with a very racially mixed population and a history of political activism) and three of them were arrested and taken to the police station. Max described the very frightening events that took place there, being left locked up for hours, not being allowed to contact his mother, and threats and some bullying questioning by detectives.

As I listened to his account, which was given extremely slowly and in detail, and with no hint of the outcome until the story was completed, I was invaded by anxiety about his treatment at the police station. I felt afraid that he was going to reveal ill treatment. I also felt righteous indignation at the indignity and absurdity of the proceedings and full of suspicion that this technical offence (fly-posting) was being utilised as an excuse to arrest and harass young black activists. I might have felt this on my own account on hearing such a story, but the extremely intense feelings aroused in me made me suspect that I was carrying a double load, my own response plus Max's unmentioned anxiety about the treatment of black people in police stations in the middle of the night. He made no reference whatever to his colour, or to the impact it must have had at the police station when his white middle class mother finally appeared the following morning to take him home!

The first indications of his capacity to openly acknowledge interest in his ethnicity came some while later when he decided to have his long hair plaited at a shop in Brixton (a part of London with a large Afro-Caribbean population). He had often played with strands of hair in sessions, pulling out the tight curls to full length and then winding them round his fingers rather in the way that young children often play with their hair, or babies play with their mothers' hair, and not at all in the way that adolescents self-consciously groom themselves. One week he told me about an abortive visit to get his hair done when he had misjudged the journey, got lost, and arrived too late. He conveyed a picture of a lost little boy wandering in Brixton, and I again felt anxious on his behalf and found it very painful to realise that he had no one to go with. When he did get his hair done, what he wanted to tell me about was how much it had hurt, how much it had cost, and how many hours it took. In fact, he said, his head was still hurting because of the hair being pulled so tight. He looked that day like a child who has had an unwanted hairstyle inflicted on him, not an adolescent, proud and challenging, testing out a Rasta identification.

It was only towards the end of his second year of therapy that he mustered any energy to explore racial difference. He had continued to provide me with evidence of its importance, for example by joining a black student centre at his college. But any exploratory remarks by me were left well alone, and there was a complete denial that it was of any interest to him that the two of us were a different colour. I could not find any way to explore the idea that he might have feelings about the difference in our experience of the world on this dimension, and I was made to feel quite stupid for bringing in such irrelevancies. He never made it clear what colour skin his girl friends had, yet assumed I knew these details, and when I would

41

discuss what it meant that he left me in the dark and then implied that he had told me all the time, the matter would be passed over. The medium for his ultimate awakening interest was his artwork, to which he devoted a lot of time. He described to me paintings and sculptures he was working on which were linked with African art, and this development reached a climax when he brought his whole Baccalaureate folder to show me his art project, which centred on the artist Diego Rivera and included many self-portraits drawing attention to his own Caribbean characteristics. There was also some eloquent writing by Max about black faces, and carefully transcribed quotations in which he seemed to place himself in a tradition of black artists exploring their bodies with pride, aware of the denigrated images whose hegemony they were disputing.

Clinical material

I should like now to describe material from sessions of the last six months of our work together. By this time (after two and half years' work) there was a sense of conviction about the relevance of my interpretations of the transference relationship. This followed a long period of blankness, in which Max seemed to absorb intellectually the links I made but then to say something amounting to "so what?", which sometimes made me feel that he needed me to say more than I yet could, and sometimes made me feel squashed.

At this time, Max was involved in exploring his homosexuality and was very eager to talk about this. He began one session by talking about a conversation with Jake, a recent lover who had suddenly ended their relationship. They had ended up feeling they were friends, he said. There was no feeling in his toneless voice. He went on to talk about a one-night stand with another man and said, "I didn't seem to feel anything about it". I commented on his speaking in a far-away fashion about events, which seemed as if they ought to have emotional significance. He returned to the topic of Jake and said he felt nothing for him either. Jake wanted the relationship to restart, but Max had said they should just be friends or they would end up hating each other. He spoke in a chilly and dismissive way about Jake but ended by remarking that it seemed cruel maybe, when Jake was feeling so involved and had said he loved him. In fact, he added, a little complacently, two people had recently said to him that they had never felt so strongly for anyone as for him, which he could not understand at all. I said that he was introducing us to a very cold part of himself that felt devoid of feeling and that he was worried that something cruel was going on when the other person felt so strongly and he felt nothing. At first Max seemed not to follow this, and he asked what I meant. When I remained silent, wondering within myself if he was indeed as uncomprehending as he appeared, he eventually suggested that perhaps I meant a cold part of his character, to which I agreed. He said that it was not so much that he felt cold, more that he felt nothing at all. "Empty?" I wondered. Mm, he responded. He then said more about Jake, who was the manager of a gay pub, and about the one-night stand, saying that he felt a bit guilty, but there was really no hurt on either side and they both knew it would be like that. As he talked, he was pulling his curls. I found myself thinking about his natural father, perhaps the original one-night stand in Max's life, and feeling very worried about risks he might be taking in relation to HIV/AIDS which at this time was at its height. In other words, I was at this point stirred up, full of painful anxiety, while he apparently remained ultra cool.

He then said this was like the situation between himself and his mother. She gets so upset, and he seems to feel nothing. I suggested that this recurrent theme of one person dead to feeling while the other felt overwhelmed perhaps had resonance for him. He asked what this word resonance meant and I explained in terms of echo, and he then agreed. (There were occasional examples of his not understanding words I would have expected to be part of his sophisticated vocabulary. I think they were probably words used in relation to metaphor, and I suspect they may have been words which I felt I had chosen rather precisely. Was this a way in which he asserted difference and distance from my cultural background, I sometimes wondered?)

I asked if he could give me an example of what he was thinking of between him and his mother. After a moment, he began to tell me a story. A few months ago, for Mother's Day, Joe (his mother's partner) gave him £10 to buy her a present. He himself had a little money too. He went to Swiss Cottage market, which is close to the Tavistock. There he saw a bag – that one, he said, pointing to his heavy rather old-fashioned brief case – and he felt he *had* to buy it. He was thinking of himself as the history student, going to university, and needing to carry his history around in a bag like that one. It cost £10. So he bought it with Joe's £10. Then he bought his mother a little box of sweets. When he got back he told Joe who was angry and demanded his money back. So Max said OK . . . at this point in the story he paused and said . . . "Oh! This is getting embarrassing when I remember what I did", and he almost squirmed. But he continued:

> I took my mother's card and went to the cash point and got the money to give to Joe. Later, when I told her what I had done and said I would pay it back, there was a tremendous row. She and Joe were very upset and angry.

I said something important had happened while he was telling me this, because he had come to feel something quite strongly at the moment when he spoke of his embarrassment, and so he was no longer the person who felt nothing. He acknowledged this. Then when he seemed about to recount another incident, I said I thought we should pause to think over what he had been telling me, which I considered important. I spoke about Joe as a father-person who he felt was helping him to do something nice for Mother; and about his own overwhelming sense of immediate need for the bag, an impulse like a very little boy's urgent need for something, like a child wanting sweets maybe. I explored the idea of the bag he needed to hold his history as a reference to his own personal past as well as to his academic interest. Max then wondered if his plan to study history was meant to help him recover from his own history. I said we could explore that idea together and then I spoke of the reversal in this incident – he gets the big and grown-up gift but Mother got the sweets. Like a little girl, he mused. I went on – "It must feel hard to be the child who wants or needs something and doesn't have resources. He would prefer to be the grown-up who could evade such disappointments", I suggested. He spoke about a belief that grown-ups ought to be strong and have their feet on the ground, but his experience was that they often didn't and he felt he was more grown-up than they. I said that in telling me the story he had felt that he had been able to face his own little child feeling of shame about his behaviour because he felt me to be a feet-on-the-ground grown-up who would not be filled with desperate feelings or become very upset or angry with him, but would be able to talk to him about the deprived little boy part of himself that felt he had nothing and could not bear someone else to have anything. He said did I mean jealousy, and I agreed that it was a kind of jealousy.

Then he began to tell me that last Friday he had cooked supper for Mum and Joe. He plans now to do this every Friday – he wants to learn to cook properly – for them and anyone else who is there. He had to go shopping first. It was a vegetarian meal, but it was a real success and he felt very good about it. I commented on his almost for the first time referring to his mother as "Mum", a warm and affectionate link instead of his usual chilly and formal references to "my mother". He expressed intense surprise at my observation. I suggested that his wish to be able to do Mum-like things such as cooking a meal that people would enjoy, that would give pleasure, was linked with his having changed in the session today – the cold part of him being counter-balanced by a much warmer part that is feeling linked with a Mum-me that has hopes of his learning things, coming alive to feelings, warming up. A bit uncertainly he asked, "Is that how you see it?" I talked of his wondering whether I had been able to keep alive hopes of his blossoming over time. He recalled often being called a zombie between the ages of 14 to 16. He had always had a serious expression and never expressed any feelings. He so admires people who can express feelings. Now he thinks there is a difference between childish and child-like. His mother and sister are child-like, can get really angry and can really laugh, but he finds it so hard. What he thinks now is that the childish thing is to button up feelings and that it is better to be able to express things. I said he felt happy about being able to face his little-boy shame and find the courage to go through the whole story with me and not suppress it, that he felt upset with himself but more alive. He then (it was almost time to stop now) spoke of how nice it was with his one-night stand which was the night after this supper; it felt so good. I felt appalled, chilled to the bone and felt this to be a terrible assault on his relations with his family and on our intimacy within the session. I said to him that he was equating the good supper and the one-night stand but that I did not think this was quite right. It seemed to me that the warmer hopeful supper was representing his hopeful, more generous, not-empty self and that the unfeeling sex gave him a place to put the cold and cruel part of himself. This was now linked to the end of the session which made him feel shut out and worried about losing contact with his more lively feelings. Max said, in a huge generalisation, a ghastly parody of psychoanalytic interpretation, "It seems that there is a pessimistic part of me as well". I pointed out that the generalisation seemed to have taken the life out of what I had said and would leave him with a platitude, not a meaningful description.

This very important exchange was taken up again in the following sessions, as he had become interested in the idea of some basic things missing in him.

He gave examples of what he thought was missing – not understanding mathematical concepts, not being able to sustain relationships nor to live out his political commitment. He linked this also with his incapacity to do life drawing in art. This led him on to talk about the beautiful model they had been asked to draw. He spoke at length about watching her dress, their exchange of looks, and his fascination and excitement as he watched her go out. Then he added that of course there is something more with a man, something extra. I suggested to him that he was showing us how he turns away and attacks his admiration and interest and the object of his desire at the moment of losing it – as the girl leaves the room, and now as we come to the end of the sessions and he sees me as departing. He was thoughtful and said, "That is very complex".

Material of this kind made it clear that his homosexual feelings were much stirred up by any loss of a woman's attention, and that his excitement about men was intended as a reproach and punishment of any woman who exposed him to fears of abandonment.

Ending therapy

A crisis arose in the middle of the last term's work. Max was completing a Foundation art course, which he had chosen to do for a year after leaving school and before going to university to study history. This had in fact been a creative solution to his typical uncertainty about choosing – he had for a long time worried how not to choose one subject at the expense of the others and then feel there had been a betrayal. He had managed in this way to make space for both enthusiasms, perhaps hinting at the growth of a sense of an internal parental couple who could make space for each other. However, he would be leaving London in September for his university course, and therapy would be ending, as he would be studying a long way away. In the middle of the term he began to talk of leaving London as soon as the art school term ended, thus missing the last month of therapy. This was an extreme repetition of the familiar pattern of pre-holiday absences, but this time it was being talked about, and I could tackle his need to leave first, and his anxieties about whether there could ever be a good ending in his life. He was able to listen and understand, and said after a lot of work that he would stay on for July. The straightforwardness with which he announced this change of mind was as big a change as the change of plan, for it acknowledged directly: "Something has happened between us in the session today and it makes a difference". His stance of arrogant cynicism seemed truly to be on the wane.

This was consolidated the following week when he talked about how much he was missing his parents who had gone on holiday, his sadness that they would not be able to come to the opening of the art college exhibition where his work was displayed, and his pleasure in his changed relationship to his sister to whom he now felt very close. No longer was he the second-class child, forever on the edge of the proper family children who "look right". He spoke of her two-year relationship with a boyfriend in contrast to his incapacity to make anything last, and we discussed her tolerance for ups and downs in comparison with his all or nothing approach. I linked these extreme states of alternating involvement and total disinterest with his feelings about what he perceived of his mother's state when he was little. I was thinking of the likely mood-cycle associated with drug use. He was amazed but not incredulous at this link and when I elaborated my interpretation seemed fascinated. This led to two memories of childhood, a very rare event.

The first was of himself on the run with his mother. They were at the beach with friends, and mother was teaching him to swim. It was wonderful, but they were waiting all the time for the police because he was supposed to be living with his adoptive family. The police broke down the door and took him back. After that he saw less of his mother and then he came to England and saw even less of her. I talked to him about his difficulty in believing that a feeling of happiness can ever be trusted to go on and how this helps us to understand why he is so drawn to make a getaway first; we both know that he had felt strongly that it would be better not to stay on here until the end. Max responded with another memory. He and his mother were at Sean's flat. (Sean was one of Mother's boyfriends when Max was two to three years old.) Mother was provoking Sean, wanting a fight, he knew that. She knocked over a glass, Sean got

47

angry, and Max remembers wanting to get out of the room, as he knew there would be violence. He can remember Sean on top of Mother and they were having sex — Mother told Sean to be careful; something to do with her menstrual blood. He was in a chair, trying to turn himself into a ball, eyes closed. We talked about his little boy muddles between sex and fighting, not knowing what it was he did not want to see, and his sense of there being no one there when he was small to notice his upset and fear. It now felt important to share with me these confused and terrifying images. Right at the end of our work together I suggested these early memories are coming alive for him because he now has a hope that coming close does not have to be so mixed up with anger and cruelty as he had believed.

In the penultimate session Max talked about a picture he had painted and named "Cutting the umbilical cord to the family". There were many associations to this, but it seemed to suggest that the cord could be cut because the infant was now viable, ready for life outside the womb, the family, and the therapy. This infant has a family and it was now clearly the adoptive family that provided this sense of belonging. Having found his family, he can begin to tackle separating from it. These new notions of proper connectedness were repeatedly threatened by the cynical "so what?" part of Max which popped up whenever separation loomed, and it was clear that this would be an ongoing point of vulnerability for him.

In the last session, for the first time in three years, Max talked about his first experience of therapy:

> When I was with Dr K. I had a drawer of toys just for me, paints and things. I remember some sessions when I just threw things all over the room, and she was left to clear them up at the end.

We explored the way that art-materials have now become very important in his ideas about how he will keep in touch with himself, because his art enables him to express and sort things out, not just hurl things round. This time he has not left me to do all the clearing up of his emotional mess by walking off. Later, he said,

> It was different with Dr K. When I stopped coming, it was chaos. My father left, I was very difficult with my mother, there were rows all the time. But then I came back here and these three years have been good.

Discussion

I would like to attempt to clarify what I think was happening to Max's sense of identity over this period. Identity is based at depth on the inner pattern of our identifications, our relationship to our internal objects in psychoanalytic terms. Therapy provided Max with the possibility of reworking these identifications and this made possible different relationships in his current life at home and elsewhere. Max, like all adopted children, has the additional complexity that the relationship to the natural parents is part of the picture. He had felt part of two quite different families. In one, the natural family, Max saw Mother as unable to take care of him or herself and Father as either absent and even completely unaware of his existence, or unreliable because of violence towards mother. He had retained links with the wider natural family including his grandparents, and this contact eventually helped him alongside the work in therapy to sort out the reality of where he belonged. In the other family, his adoptive family, Mother was reliable but was felt to prefer her own children, and Father was seen as critical and abandoning. The increased approach to Joe was external evidence of the growth of a more benign inner father figure.

Max's evolving sexual identity was profoundly influenced by these perceptions. His homosexual side expresses his fear of cruel heterosexuality. He was always afraid that intercourse would lead to pregnancy for which there was no readiness and that a girl would trap him into responsibilities he could not manage. Thus there would be a repetition of a mother who could not care for her baby and a father who would abandon them. But his homosexual leanings also contained elements of masochistic submission which put him in danger, and this was due to his identification with his abused mother who was addicted to abuse, through sex and drugs. When we ended work, the balance of homosexual and heterosexual trends remained very fluid, but Max had some grasp of the emotional dynamics at work in these choices, and in the oscillation between his more narcissistic preoccupations and his growing capacity for interest in others. My work was aimed at elucidating the basis of his sexual feelings, and exploring his underlying conflict in terms of whether his approach to a sexual partner was rooted in loving or hating feelings towards himself and the other.

The surprising development in the last term of his capacity for imaginative links, which countered the "so what?" part of his personality, was linked to the recovery of lost memories, and many holes thus being filled in. Instead of a mind which easily dropped things, on the model of his mother's mind impaired by drugs, there was a sense of quite a well-functioning mind, which could gather and store his thoughts and memories, and reflect on them. The improvement in his mental functioning appeared initially in his academic work, and involved his resisting the idea of being second-rate, the one who has to fail and to experience denigration at the hands of his successful siblings. In the last sessions, this new capacity for thought became linked to emotional experience. What it felt like in the room was that we had each acquired an extra dimension. I had earlier often felt denuded and stripped of human qualities by his incomprehension of emotional meaningfulness.

As we said goodbye, I noticed that the boy who had been tormented by not knowing what to wear, and who had tried a dozen hairstyles, looked comfortable in his clothes, had a haircut that suited him and was a good-looking young man.

Conclusion

The opportunity for further work in later adolescence was important in freeing Max to find a way of living which was less over-determined by his self-crippling defences. The need to rework the meaning of loss of birth parents and entry into an adoptive family recurrently throughout life is an unavoidable task for all adoptees. Finding the place where one fits within such a complex network of love, let-down, loss, and second chance is always difficult. Other points of potential crises include the birth of children in the next generation. But perhaps the adolescent tasks of separation, establishment of sexual relationships, and the entry into adult responsibilities are the toughest time of all. In the inner world the first separation has been imbued with catastrophe, sexual partnerships are felt to be damaging to both parties and a threat to a potential baby, and there are ties to parental figures unable to shoulder the work of adulthood. The pain of relinquishing the early damaged and damaging inner parental figures in order to find a life for oneself can be very great. I think it is here that psychotherapy has so much to offer.

Max's development during his therapy seems to me to provide a vivid example of the way that the shaping of identity in an adolescent is rooted in the nature of internal object relations and in particular to allow us to think about how adolescent sexual development depends on the young person's unconscious perception of the parental couple.

3

RIGIDITY AND STABILITY IN A PSYCHOTIC PATIENT

Some thoughts about obstacles to facing reality in psychotherapy (1997)

This chapter is an attempt to think about a particular kind of rigidity in a post-autistic patient who lives simultaneously in a psychotic private world and in the world of relationships and shared meanings. I worked with Holly for nine years and shall discuss the material of a session some months prior to the end of her therapy. In considering the meaning of our interchange I wish to distinguish between the changes that have been achieved and the ongoing obsessional ruminative power of the psychotic process. I shall try to consider these from two perspectives: the patient's continuing partial addiction to delusional defensive structures, which she experiences as protective, and the analyst's countertransference difficulties in facing the limitations of the work. Both of us needed to struggle with anxieties about facing reality; the reality of the approaching end of the treatment brought these into clearer focus.

I shall begin with some details of the patient's history. She is the first child of a middle-class couple and is now 22 years old. She has a sister three years younger than herself. When I met her parents to explore the possibility of Holly beginning psychotherapy, they told me with the most intense outpouring of feelings about her early life. The pregnancy had gone well, and Mother was waiting with happy anticipation for the arrival of a much-wanted baby. This mood was massively

DOI: 10.4324/9781003325543-5

disrupted by what seems to have been a traumatic experience of labour and child birth, when Mother felt overwhelmed by pain, and unsupported and criticised by medical and nursing staff. After a very long labour, Holly was delivered by forceps and said to be at risk; the parents felt this was due to oxygen deficiency, but the details are not clear.

The baby was not given to Mother to hold but nursed initially in intensive care. Subsequently breast-feeding was established and continued for three months. The outstanding memories of the early months which Mother communicated were two – firstly, the sense that whatever she did for Holly, the baby cried. She could not satisfy or calm her and felt persecuted by the baby's distress. As in the hospital at the birth, she felt criticised and found wanting as a mother. The baby's misery was not something she could take in and bear, but a source of persecution. She told me, with startling and moving honesty, that there was something I needed to know from the start: 'You will never understand Holly unless you bear in mind that I hated her. I feel guilty about this, but I really did hate her.' She went on to describe a second crucial event which occurred when she showed the new baby to her own mother. Here I need to include some of the history of Mother's family of origin; she herself is the younger of two sisters. Her older sister, Jane, was a severely autistic child who began to deteriorate markedly at age twelve and has been institutionalised since then. Grandmother looked at the new baby and said, 'Good heavens! It's Jane.' I do not know whether Holly did resemble Jane, but what this remark heralded was a difficult struggle between Mother and Grandmother over how to treat Holly, and it aroused acute terror in Mother that this baby would indeed have a similar history.

Holly cried less after breast-feeding was abandoned and found solace in playing on her own for hours at a time. She showed very little interest in her parents or anyone else. Mother's sense of rejection and uselessness increased. At an early developmental check, deafness was suggested, but this turned out to be a false trail. Mother was terribly worried about Holly and tried to get her anxieties taken seriously. It is hard retrospectively to understand the absence of professional concern about Holly, but what probably played a part was that Mother's own intense anxiety, guilt and upset was so palpable. She seems to have felt trapped between a kind husband who tried to reassure her by dwelling on all positive signs in Holly's development and her own mother, who was committed to the notion that history was repeating itself.

When Holly was two the family consulted a child psychiatrist because of her peculiar language development – instead of responding or replying, she would repeat what was said to her. He advised treatment for Mother, and this was arranged. Nearly two years later, on seeing Holly for review, he was very alarmed and said help for Holly was now urgently required. The family was referred to a hospital for psychotic children quite some distance from their home. Holly, Mother and her younger sister Caroline, aged one, were admitted together. After a brief time, Mother and Caroline returned home and Holly remained an in-patient for a further seven months with weekends at home. She was diagnosed at this time as autistic. I heard many terrifying memories of her time in hospital during her therapy. My overall impression was that she may have experienced chronic emotional abuse from the staff. Certainly Holly was driven mad with terror. For years this revived when approaching any break in therapy which she would experience as my sending her back to the hospital.

When she returned home, she was placed in a small school for autistic children. Holly herself gained a good deal from this school, and by the time she was 11 years old she progressed to be able to manage three and a half days a week in mainstream primary school, with children one year younger than herself. However, Mother was extremely upset by the attitude of the special school staff who, she felt, viewed mothers as responsible for their children's autistic condition. The active involvement demanded of the parents was thus a torture to her. When the school had to close down, there was a crisis about Holly's future education since mainstream secondary school on a full-time basis was clearly not an option. Eventually she was placed in a school for children with moderate learning difficulties, and when I became involved this placement was at risk since Holly was very difficult to manage in a class of low I.Q. but otherwise fairly ordinary children. As I came to realise, Holly was being subjected to verbal and sexual abuse by the other children and had retreated behind a non-stop flow of psychotic talk which was driving the teachers mad with frustration.

A brief account of the therapy

When I began to see Holly, I encountered a completely mad child. She never stopped speaking, but it was possible to detect in the flow of crazy talk that she had hopes of me. She communicated a desperate

54

wish that I might be able to bear her projections and an intense fear that she would be too much for me as she felt she had been for everyone else. I was shocked at the bizarre discrepancy between what she herself memorably described as 'verbal diarrhoea', a flood of words with frequent bodily references and confusion of body parts, and her actual physical presence. She looked uncannily like her mother, with the same hairstyle, and even shared a similar ultra middle-class tone of voice though with added decibels and a disconcerting absence of range. She had a sophisticated vocabulary and an additional private language to refer to her 'autistic objects' (Tustin, 1981). She always carried with her a bag full of small items to which she gave idiosyncratic meanings. For example, she called the empty boxes which usually house camera films 'cylinders', an entirely accurate correct description of their shape, but to her the reference was to faecal stool. For years she held in each hand throughout her sessions one or other of these precious objects, which she said were her protectors. Her awareness of the need for protection of the vulnerable parts of the self seemed an indication of her preconception (Bion, 1962b) of the protective function of a good object and her need to locate such an object. Much later, when she discovered she had bones and thus an internal structure which did not melt when she was flooded with emotion, she was able to leave her bag closed on the table, and eventually to lie on the couch for her sessions.

She lived a life of terror – of falling to pieces, fragmenting in body or mind, and desperately trying to protect herself from a cruelly invasive object which was intent on wounding her. She always wore trousers because she needed the reassurance of layers of clothing over her vagina and anus to prevent hostile assault. For a long time, she insisted that she possessed a penis (she constructed hundreds of phallic models, for example of lighthouses or windmills, to represent this). Eventually, she could talk to me about her dread of the 'hole', of being and having nothing if she gave up this delusional penis. She could not bear contact with her mother and never used female nouns or pronouns during this period. Eventually she was able to acknowledge her femininity and have a much warmer relationship with her mother.

The most important thread of her therapy was the wish to drive me mad and thus rid herself of the unbearable psychological pain and confusion of feeling mad herself, and the simultaneous hope that I would survive this onslaught. For the first year or so, I spent virtually whole sessions with no idea of what was going on. The one thing I could reliably manage was to maintain the setting of the beginning and end of the session. Sometimes I could observe and describe meaningful sequences and we could have a conversation, but at other times the bombardment of nonsense was so exhausting that I was dulled into virtual inactivity or stale repetition of interpretations which had previously meant something. I felt immured in the atmosphere of a hospital ward for severe schizophrenics without the benefit of medication.

When I realised that the point was to test my sanity, Holly became able to tell me with flagrant enjoyment that she was trying to drive me potty. An infinite variety of formulations appeared: 'I want to drive you crazy, up the wall, round the bend', etc. Her usual method was to indulge in verbal masturbation. She quickly understood this idea, and spoke about 'rubbing with my words.' However, this initial understanding did little to abate her frantic activity when she was anxious.

Over time there was a lessening of her haunting terrors, which she had spent a lifetime avoiding through obsessional rituals and thoughts. One such manoeuvre was to 'close the doors in my ears' which she would act out when she did not want to hear what I was saying. As the conviction that I was not to be trusted and would abandon her was replaced by a growing belief in my truthfulness – I seemed not to forget her, to return after holidays as promised etc. – so the need to close her ears to reality receded. The working through of these persecutory anxieties in her therapy enabled her to reduce her interminable efforts to control the members of her family. This lessening of omnipotent control allowed a more normal family life to develop. The terror she felt at each tiny step towards relaxing her omnipotence was extreme, and for years the family felt constrained by the fear of evoking her frightening tantrums. She once tried to force me to accept a ring from her on my wedding ring finger (she felt she could thus bind me to her as if in marriage) and when I did not allow her to do this she was distraught with rage and fear.

When Holly was 18, plans had to be made for her future. When she left the school for autistic children, the only local possibility was for her to attend a work-centre for learning disabled adults and to live at home. This was unsuitable, since the family, especially her younger sister, needed some opportunity for ordinary life, and Holly needed support for further social development. Most fortunately, an unusual place was found. An ordered, humane and down-to-earth institution with good community links offered her a long-term home. It was agreed that Holly could be brought for continuing therapy once a week. Holly could attend further education classes and be part of a large community where she became liked and respected. She is on the residents' committee, and is not seen as a mad person at all. The contrast between the Holly I know and Holly 'the resident' is quite dramatic.

Introduction to the session

This is the last session before an Easter holiday and it is planned to end the therapy in the summer. This decision was made by me and was something Holly seemed to understand. She seemed able to tolerate it as an idea as long as we could speak about her wish to keep in touch with me from time to time. She felt this link to an external Mrs Rustin would keep alive what she called 'the inside Mrs Rustin' with whom she often had conversations. Perhaps it was also felt to keep alive the importance and reality of her experience of madness which she had shared so starkly with me. In the last period of a long analysis, there is often a revisiting of old themes.

With Holly this process has had the effect of making me feel full of doubt about how much has been achieved. Sometimes it seems I have only succeeded in helping her to elaborate fundamentally narcissistic structures, which do enable her to function with less anxiety and in more socially acceptable ways, but which also render her very difficult to reach. The energy required to go on with the struggle to draw her out of her retreat (Steiner, 1993) and into more lively contact with reality is phenomenal. This is true both with reference to her internal reality, her contact with emotional experiences, and to external reality. In the session to be discussed I attempt to speak to her from outside the ongoing psychotic flow which occupies so much of her mental space.

As a preliminary, I would like to explain some references in the material. First, the people Holly speaks about. Gwen was her key worker when she first went to live away from home. When Gwen became pregnant she left her work, so she represents Holly's anxiety about being abandoned in favour of another baby. Maureen, an older woman of very calm temperament, replaced Gwen. She is extremely important to Holly, who discovered the quality of 'motherliness' in

Maureen. Holly is possessive of Maureen and believes that she and Maureen will always live in the same house. Granny is a sinister figure from the point of view of her prospects for psychic change. In reality, her grandmother indulges Holly's obsessions, and tends to blame everyone else for Holly's problems. In Holly's internal world she is an ally in all her masturbatory phantasies as Granny is always in favour of the avoidance of mental pain. Sally is one of the older women who accompany Holly to the Clinic. The muffin man is a character in a children's song – 'Do you know the muffin man?' – and has become a fixture in her imagination, representing the idea of a man who would protect her against the terrifying anxieties aroused by anything female. He is a man who can feed her muffins and sweets, and help her to avoid contact with the feeding breast.

Holly uses some private words in this session. I understand the meaning of these as follows:

1   A 'shuddle' is a masturbatory phallic object which has the qualities of a shuttle (always moving), of muddle, of shit, and of shuddering or shivering with dread.
2   A 'wally' in children's slang is someone stupid, out-of-touch – this word is used as a form of abuse of other people. For Holly there are many types of wally and she is very frightened of them, especially brown or black wallies. She has no doubt heard other children call her a wally.
3   A 'wibble' has reference to a nipple-penis confusion, to an intrusive object, and one which is wibbly-wobbly, that is, in permanent motion, unstable and excited.
4   A 'hamihocker' – these are the most frightening creatures in Holly's dreams and phantasies. Her perception of the external world used to be full of hamihockers. They now occur only in her dreams. They have a quality of ruthless machines, with an intention to hurt her. They are very complicated conceptions, somewhat like Bion's idea of 'bizarre objects' (Bion, 1957). They are conglomerates of persecutory fragments.

The session

In the corridor on the way to my room Holly said, 'The shuddle made me laugh in the toilet. I was worried he would pick me up, and poke my bottom.' When she lay on the couch she added, 'Gwen

58

was like a shuddle when she was my key-worker.' I said, she wanted me to know she was frightened. This was the last session of the term and this is the last holiday before she stops coming to the Clinic to see me. She is worried that I am going to turn into a Gwen-person in her mind who is hurting her by leaving her to look after another baby. 'Mm. That's it,' Holly said.

> Yesterday in the café Jane told me off. The strange man upset me. He took no notice. I said "Please may I have a cream carton" [repeats *sotto voce*] and he did not listen. I was going on and on. He was Mr Rustin. He was an ignoring Daddy.

After a brief pause she added, 'I've come to talk to you.' I said that she felt that the Daddy aspect of Mrs Rustin was not listening and understanding how hard it was for her not to go on having therapy every week, like more and more cream cartons, but that she hoped that she could talk to me about this problem of not feeling understood. Holly said, 'He told me not to ask silly questions. The strange man mocked me.' I said that she felt mocked instead of understood, but that she hoped to find in me a Daddy who could think about her endless desire for milk. 'That's right.'

Holly went on 'Maureen (present key-worker) told me to pack it in. The man made me miserable.' I said she was miserable that this was the last session this term. 'Maureen made remarks about me.' I said she was letting me know that even Maureen gets fed up with her sometimes, and she is worried that I do too. 'It was at McDonald's. Maureen made me feel offended. She made me blush. She made me feel pink. She made me red in the face. . . . I love Maureen O'Dowd. In the restaurant I laughed about the yellow potty-boat. The Granny-boat.' Holly giggled and imitated a sickly-sweet old lady cooing over a baby. 'The black man reminds me of a shuddle.' I said she was preferring to be mad now instead of sad. Holly replied, 'Yesterday I was kissing the skeleton spoon.' I said she was agreeing with me: she wanted to pretend that frightening ideas about dying, and specially about the Mrs Rustin inside her turning into a skeleton, could be turned into an exciting joke. Holly responded, 'I like the bottom of a yoghurt carton and saying I'm not a magician.' I said that she often tried to believe she was a magician.

Holly then told me she was going home on Sunday. 'Tomorrow it will be two nights until I go home, then it will be one night, then it will be Sunday.' I said she liked to be clear, it helped her to wait. I explained that she was also thinking about the three sessions she will miss during the holidays, and that she has quite a clear picture of this in her mind, and knows that she will then be returning to see me. Holly said, 'Yes, I have a clear picture.' Pause. 'Sally told me to wait.' I said she feels everyone is expecting her to be able to wait. Holly said, 'I find it very difficult. I had to talk to Maureen.' I said she was thinking about two different ideas she has about me. Sometimes she feels I am asking her to manage something that is so difficult for her, to learn how to wait, but she is also pleased to be able to tell me about this and feel understood. Holly said, 'I've come to talk to you.' I said she was finding it helpful, and Holly replied with real feeling 'Yes, I'm finding it very helpful.'

She went on, 'The strange man made me sad.' I said she was feeling jealous of the Daddy who she felt I would be with during the holiday. 'He mocked me.' I said she was afraid of an idea of a Daddy who would laugh at her sadness. 'He had black eyes. A white nose. He was pale. I was homesick.' I said, 'You felt you had lost the friendly understanding Daddy inside you.' 'Sally told me to stop demanding. I don't like you taking away my blue spoon. I'm afraid you will throw it away.' I asked her to tell me about this spoon. 'Maureen gave it to me from Disneyland. It goes purple in the water.' I said she felt I would be jealous of something special that she had as a present from Maureen, so jealous that I would want to take it away from her. Holly explained, 'Sometimes I bang the spoon on my mouth . . . I've come to talk to you.' I talked more about her hope that I could bear her having something that she liked that was nothing to do with me, and how important it was to her to remember that Maureen is fond of her when she knows she made Maureen feel irritated with her in McDonald's.

'I'm going shopping tomorrow. I shall buy Nivea, shampoo, bubble bath. Then next time I shall buy spoons, white ones to play with. I play with them in my hospital. I give myself a tonic. I'm going to buy toothpaste on Saturday.' I said she had lots of ideas about how to look after herself during the holiday. 'I shall be nice and clean and look pretty.'

'I dreamt about the yellow potty in the passage way. The music made me laugh. It reminded me about the muffin man who I held onto when I was little.' I said there were different ways of holding on: old ways, like in her dream, and new ways like the plans to take care of herself and think about the part of her that wanted to get better and stronger. Holly said, 'like holding on to the melamine round the thermos that I got from Mummy.' I said she was thinking about her different ways of holding on. Holly continued: 'Going back to square one. Using the base of a yoghurt carton as a shuddle. The red pointer I was scared of, digging into me. It was wibble shaped.'

I said she understands that her old ways of holding on hurt her, were not good for her. The new ways make her feel better.

> In my dream I held the pointer to stop it digging into me. The bird was in my dream. I want to kiss the black bird that flies. I use the yoghurt carton as a pet, a bird, and I kiss it. I think that kissing the yoghurt carton is a joke.

I said she was getting into a muddle now. Holly went on 'I use it as a nipple. I kiss it and say "you said the creed." It's perfectly natural.' This last phrase was uttered in a different voice and I asked whose voice it was. Holly replied, 'I want to trick you.' I said the trick was to get things in a muddle. Holly continued, 'I use it as food . . . as a hamihocker, as a foot.' I said she was showing me that the trick is that a bit of plastic can be made into anything she fancies in her mind, there is then no difference between anything at all. Holly said, 'The noise in the distance reminds me of a creamy white wally. I want to rub on the white wally. But the grey wally scares me.' I said she knew that all these imaginary things changed quickly in her mind, that she could not get hold of anything solid to keep herself feeling safe. 'They turn into shuddles that frighten me. When Maureen is my key worker I rub on the shuddle. I want you to do that and be the same as me and get excited.' I said she wanted me to be lonely like her, not to have a Daddy to be with, so that I would really understand why she tries to rub away her unhappiness. Holly added, 'I want to comfort in my bottom. I kiss the shuddle in my dream. Then it smells of my bottom.'

I said we were near the end of the session now and that Holly was trying to distract herself from her sad feelings, and that we both knew that when she filled up her mind with these bottom-thoughts it was hard for her to think of anything else. I wondered if there was anything she could do about it. 'Clear it up,' she said. I wondered if she wanted to. 'I want a window catch to let the fresh air in. It will take the stale smells away.' I said she was tired of the old stuff. Holly said, 'I am. I am tired of shit as well. I want fresh air instead of shit. Shit makes me sick. The man of shit kicks me inside me and makes me feel sick. The bottom man. The chocolate man.' I said she was telling me that her faeces in her bottom have sometimes felt to her to be just like a penis and this idea made her feel very muddled. 'Black men and children remind me of shit.' I said she was afraid that I was sick of her and would only remember the messy, muddled Holly. She replied, 'I've come to talk to you.' I said she now believes I could also keep the other aspects of Holly alive in my mind. 'I don't like going back to the shuddle.' I said she was afraid of the part of her that creates muddle and terror. 'I've got the base of a yoghurt carton at the convent. I find it unbelievable! (shouted) I want it to be a bosom. I shove it on my mouth.'

I said she did not believe it actually was. It was very painful for her when at the end of the session she felt that I was the mother she needed who had good things that could feed her in my mind. Now it was time for us to stop. Holly said goodbye as she left. This is not a very frequent occurrence.

Discussion

This session reveals forces in conflict in Holly's mind. There are moments of contact with creative potential but also evident is the power of the undertow of her autistic and psychotic thinking. Keeping her feet on the ground, being grounded in reality, is extremely difficult for her to sustain because it involves so much pain, but in this session there are a number of moments in which she moves towards reality. The many references to colours in Holly's associations might be considered an indication of her growing interest in distinctions and potential transformations, and her growing awareness of ambivalence in contrast to extreme splitting between good and bad. Images of hope in her material have been sustaining to me, in contrast to her attacks on either of us being able to see something good or beautiful. She has a recurrent phantasy of taking my eyes out of their sockets so that all I would see would be dark emptiness. This is a terrible but clear description of her attempts to destroy my hope.

At the beginning of the session we are on familiar territory. She resorts to the shuddle to deaden feelings and projects disgust and despair into me, which is intended to obscure from herself and me her anxieties about loss. When this situation is contained, she goes on to speak about her possessiveness and greed. I have a vivid image of a bowlful of little cartons of cream, and of Holly's desire for the whole lot. Also implicit is the problem she has of getting stuck on one particular thing, the need for sameness and repetition. This is a continuing difficulty for her parents, who try to introduce her to new experiences, while Holly demands always to have the same food (scrambled eggs, chocolate pudding, etc.) and the same treats (going for a bus ride to a place where she can go shopping for smooth round objects of some kind) and the same conversation (she bullies her mother to speak the script she provides and Mother needs a lot of courage to deviate from this). In important contrast to this passion for repeating something comfortingly familiar is the reference to the strange man. This is the strangeness of the unknown, which stimulates in Holly not curiosity and interest, but panic. She projects her harshly critical superego into the man. On this occasion I did not enquire about the reality of what had happened, but sometimes I have done, and it has become quite clear that Holly knows she is talking to me about what is going on in her mind, and can distinguish quite well between that and actual events.

The first shift in the direction of tolerating reality is when she tells me that Maureen got fed up. She has previously maintained an unpunctured idealisation of Maureen, and I registered a shock of excitement and hope as she dared to acknowledge a change. A second surprise is when I heard the everyday fact that she was in McDonald's. I do not think I have ever before been allowed to know that she has been in a particular public place, a place I too could know. We are always stuck together in a world lacking specificity of time or place; I am rarely allowed to share Holly's real life activities, and I felt a thrill to catch this glimpse.

As she struggles with the mixed emotions evoked by Maureen who has shamed her, but whom she loves, an intolerable situation develops. If she were to bring together the shame and the love, she would experience guilt which she cannot bear, so there is a defensive retreat from this threshold.

But with some support from me, she rejects the magic solution and emerges to locate herself very firmly in time. The clarity of her thinking is impressive, and there is a further development when she describes seeking help from Maureen with the problem of waiting instead of resorting to magic. This is a firm choice for dependence on an external object, which is a real and non-idealised object, and against the narcissistic evasion. This is followed by a real gift to me when she tells me I have been very helpful. Holly has felt that she has been given something good, and experiences and expresses gratitude. This is linked with being able to stay, for a few moments, in a sad rather than mad state. She is 'homesick,' in touch with missing something essential to feeling that she has a psychic home. This home is both a place in my mind and her internalised capacity to think about herself, which so often gets destroyed. The problem of mourning all that has been lost in the years of her deluded existence is frequently too much to bear, even briefly.

At this point she is more able to feel her own desire for something outside herself, and can acknowledge her demandingness. This experience is terrible for her, both because she fears overwhelming a weak object and because she has so little capacity to bear the frustration of not possessing all that she desires. So the insupportable need is projected into me, and Holly investigates, as so often before, whether I can stand such emotion.

When I made the link back to Maureen, I think this revived her hope of having the capacity to sustain her loving feelings for Maureen, but at this moment there is an explosion of envy at the creative work we have been doing together. The retreat to the yellow potty is a vicious attack on the part of herself that can take in caring capacities. The introjective identification has been quite fully experienced and the bitter disappointment and despair evoked in the dependent part of the self that is now being betrayed is projected wholesale into me.

In such circumstances, it is hard to believe in the reality of what has just been happening. The slough of despond (Bunyan's *Pilgrim's Progress*) sucks one in. I have found that to describe the destruction, which I have done many, many times, is not enough to bring about a shift. This is because Holly is no longer aware of any hope at all, but is entirely in the grip of the counter-system of narcissistic object relations, with all the false friends aiding and abetting this disavowal. So I have learnt to speak about the projected sane part of her.

I believe that my incipient mindless despair mirrors my patient's problem, and that it is my task not to become hopeless and confused, but to speak up for the temporarily abandoned, dependent infantile self. The therapist's problem, with a psychotic patient, is often echoed by the way in which parents and teachers get stuck in very low expectations and cannot remain responsive to the possibilities for change and development. Much of my work with Holly's parents has been to try to pull them out of this state of numbed passivity in the face of her illness and destructiveness.

The next part of the session illustrates Holly's struggles with psychic truth. In her dream, there is contact with reality; the bird flying away is a well-known image for us of my freedom to leave her, which hurts and threatens her. She substitutes for this the pet, the autistic object that can be manipulated in any way she wishes. But she is aware that a trick is being played. The trick is the claim that we are exactly the same, in which case she could not miss me, for I would have nothing to offer her. As the trick is elaborated, and everything is reduced to an anal world, depression wells up in me, depression about her vulnerability to psychotic delusion, and the tremendous limitations of my work. At this point, I think I felt that I could not do any more. She had to do something. But I could remind her of her capacity to make such a choice, as I did in quite an explicit way, by asking her if she could do anything about the overwhelming anal stink. The idea of fresh air has been an important discovery for her, as the image of opening a window involves a recognition that the inside world so impregnated with her rubbish can be improved by contact with an alive outside world if she allows it in.

The last minutes of the session are a tremendous struggle between her mad system of confusing, useless, manipulable things (an empty yoghurt carton – she used to have literally dozens of these at any one time) and the quality of contact she can have with a real person. She is fighting for her sanity when she protests about the unbelievable nature of this way of looking at the world, and the fight enables her to say goodbye to me because she has allowed my existence to continue after her departure.

Concluding reflections

I think Holly is always battling with the painfulness of facing what Money-Kyrle describes as 'the facts of life' (Money-Kyrle, 1968). These are three fundamental truths to be faced if we are to achieve mental stability. There is firstly the difference of the generations – adult and child, analyst and patient do not have the same responsibilities or capacities. Secondly, the difference of the sexes – male and female can have complementarity, but they are distinct. If we have the physical attributes of one sex, we must lack those of the other. Both these distinctions are a source of mental pain because they give rise to envy and jealousy. Thirdly, there is the reality of the passage of time, and our own mortality.

Holly struggled to deny the difference between herself and her parents: she tried to blot out her mother, and create a world in which there was only Daddy and herself, no mother and no sister. Externally this has greatly changed, but in the transference it has to be confronted again and again. She also tried to maintain that a delusional penis was equivalent to a real one, and that she could be a boy if she wanted. This idea too has given way to a knowledge of her longing for a boyfriend, but as in this session, there is a frequent retreat to equating faeces and penis, and thus denying difference and lack.

But perhaps most central in this final phase of work is the issue of the termination of the treatment. Time is now of the essence. We have had a lot of time together, and its coming to an end raises for both of us problems of mourning. Most urgent for Holly is the question of whether she has enough strength in the sane part of her mind to provide a continuing bulwark against madness. In particular, will she be able to forgive me enough for leaving her to remain in touch with me internally and thus converse with herself. There is the problem of the rage and envy with me when I am not her possession, and the cruelty with which she can take revenge both on me and on the part of herself that is deeply attached to me. In so far as these destructive processes unravel in our work, her stability is undermined, and she then resorts to obsessional rigidities to prevent a psychotic breakdown. These rigid structures are serviceable in a certain very limited way, but they prevent any real relationships developing, and they have their own fragilities too, since they are impervious to reality and therefore vulnerable when change forces its way into consciousness. So the question is whether she can achieve acknowledgement of the end of our work and mourn both what it has offered her, and what it cannot do. For both of us, this involves bearing my limitations. Holly has often seen me close to my wits' end. Distinguishing between what I have failed to understand or bear and what I could and did provide for her can be the basis for her continued internal contact with an imperfect but valuable object. She once told me that the inside Mrs Rustin was telling her in a horrid hissing voice that she would never come back and see her because she was 'fed up to the back teeth.' Then she acted out unlocking the doors in her ears and announced 'Now I can hear the outside Mrs Rustin.' When I asked what she could now hear she said 'You are talking sense in a kind voice.'

For the therapist of such a patient there is also a painful process to face. Therapeutic zeal or omnipotence takes a massive bashing in work of this sort although the awareness of one's dependence on one's own internal good objects to withstand the loneliness of working with a psychotic patient is both tested and deepened. My patient is still a very fragile and limited person, though she is now a human being who can give pleasure and contribute to life, and receive pleasure through relationships. She remains very vulnerable to external circumstances, which may not always be as supportive as they now are.

I think there has been a tendency for me to experience in the countertransference a reluctance to face the facts of life. The pervasive atmosphere of being in another world, not at all the same as the everyday world, created in such therapies interferes with realistic thinking. I have certainly had the idea that I could never end Holly's treatment, but that I am needed on a lifelong basis. The patient's difficulty in internalising a good object is colluded with once one starts to think that only an external analytic presence can make a difference. One is also in danger of agreeing with the patient's view that such a specially needy baby must never be faced with the reality of there being other babies to consider.

There is a particularly seductive quality in the weird understandings achieved – no-one else can make sense of the details of her rituals, for example, and this tends to generate ideas of therapeutic self-importance. There is a pressure to go on elaborating interpretations of the autistic defences and to lose sight of the need to pull the patient out of them. There is a dulling of necessary anger at the cruel waste of her life and the potential waste of the therapist's time. Holly has always made it difficult for me to mobilise my justified anger with her because she experiences resistance to her manoeuvres as physical and mental assault, and because she then attempts to twist the straight talking into a sadomasochistic exchange.

The setting for psychoanalytic therapy with its emphasis on structured reliability is a double-edged matter with such patients – the regular sessions can become part of the patient's organised evasion of life unless one is very attentive. From this point of view, it is crucial that the setting of an analysis is understood to include its termination. Working towards ending has helped me to reflect more constructively on ways in which I have sometimes been co-opted to maintain a psychotic equilibrium rather than consistently challenge it.

SECTION 2

ASSESSMENT IN CHILD PSYCHOTHERAPY

4

A CHILD PSYCHOTHERAPIST'S APPROACH TO ASSESSMENT

An introductory outline (2000)

My experience of assessing the needs of children and families for therapeutic intervention was for most of my life located in the Child and Family department of the Tavistock Clinic. This department had both a broad remit to provide psychological help to the local community and a specialist function as a national centre for psychotherapy. This meant that while there were specialist and expert resources available in the clinic, and a level of psychotherapy provision which was unusual because of both its regional and national reputation and its extensive training function, the clinical approach was one which was adaptable and relevant to local child and family services. Brief as well as more extended interventions were part of the range of work undertaken. The age range of patients extended from very young pre-school children to older adolescents.

The multidisciplinary team which became the well-established basis for NHS mental health provision for children, adolescents and their families in the second half of the twentieth century is of course differently constituted in different places. For example, nurses play a much more prominent role in in-patient facilities, and there are significant different local and regional factors despite efforts to achieve greater equality of provision. Assessment of referred cases will of course be carried out by a large variety of professionals, including psychiatrists, clinical psychologists, child psychotherapists, clinical nurse specialists, social workers and family therapists.

DOI: 10.4324/9781003325543-7

The model of work to be described is also relevant to private practice settings. The essential point is the emphasis placed on assessment of the child or young person in context, including family, nursery, school or college, peer group and the wider community. This involves recognising the importance of effective collaborative work with other relevant agencies, and means that private practitioners need to create professional structures which can sustain the necessary breadth of approach. Giving proper weight to both internal and external factors, and to child and parents, is exceptionally difficult if only one worker is available.

The purposes of assessment as conceptualised here are threefold and will be differently deployed in each individual case. Firstly, an attempt to assess whether scarce psychotherapeutic resources are likely to make a significant contribution in any particular case is unavoidable. Secondly, a psychotherapeutically informed exploration of a child's state of mind can be a valuable element within a broader-based assessment. For example, referrals may include a request from Social Services for advice about placement, or arise from concern by parents or teachers about educational issues, or be focused on the need to assess the degree of risk of self-harm or other violent behaviour. The study of the child's inner state in individual exploratory assessment sessions offers information of a different kind from that gained in other modes of assessment. The facts of the inner world complement what we can know from more external sources and the two taken together can enable us to make more solidly based decisions about what interventions are required. Thirdly, I argue that an assessment is a significant process in its own right, not just an assessment for something else, and should be viewed as a brief intervention with considerable therapeutic potential.

Winnicott's classic 'Therapeutic Consultations in Child Psychiatry' (1971) is perhaps the best-known example of such thinking. While we cannot all have the intuitive genius of Winnicott, there is ample evidence that sometimes a quite brief contact, when it gets to the heart of what matters at that moment, can facilitate a big shift. Gifted clinicians have continued to explore the potential of brief work of various kinds. Pioneers in this area have included Harris (1966); Daws (1989); Hopkins (1992); Dartington (1998). If we can create an atmosphere in which child and family feel they are being consulted by the therapist as well as seeking consultation with the therapist about what is wrong, the potential mobilisation of the capacities for thought and understanding is safeguarded. Brief work depends, crucially, on the sense of a shared task. The therapist's contribution is to supply an essential missing element which can set the process of ongoing development in individuals and families going again.

The growth of family therapy paradigms has greatly added to the range of ways in which the assessment of troubled children can be approached. There is now available an enriched understanding of the complex interconnections between an individual child's problems in living and wider family functioning. Work with whole families often plays a part in a broad assessment, and whether or not the whole family is seen together as a unit, the therapist will be trying to keep a sense of the family's shape, style and history in mind when thinking about any individual child. The family as seen in the child's mind will not be the same as the family we ourselves observe, but the two perspectives must be viewed as vertices whose divergences are of special interest. Co-work between child and family therapists was an area of significant growth and mutual discovery in the final twenty years of the last century (Kraemer, 1997; Lindsey, 1997; Reid, 1999a).

While the embeddedness of psychotherapists' assessment work in a broader professional culture needs to be emphasised, I now need to delineate some of the special features arising from our psychoanalytic psychotherapy roots. Fundamental convictions underlie the particular techniques employed in these first contacts with patients. The most important of these is that close and detailed observation is the basis for clinical understanding. This starts with observation of the use the patient makes of the setting that is offered – the relationship to the waiting room, the therapist's room, the toys and other material provided – and most importantly the relationship to the therapist herself. Where does the child choose to place himself? What does he look at? How does he respond to what the therapist says? What is the quality of his way of inhabiting his own body – restless, uncomfortable, excitable, relaxed, tense?

Child psychotherapists are trained to observe in great detail interactions between babies and young children and their carers. This naturalistic literal observation, in which judgement and attribution of meaning are kept as separate as possible, is an invaluable resource in gathering rich material in assessment sessions, and in keeping maximally open-minded. The instrument we rely on is not a mechanical one, like an x-ray machine, but, rather, our own skilled capacities for recording in the mind a large array of observations which may in due course acquire pattern and meaning as they are reflected upon. The opportunity for ongoing discussion of work in progress with experienced colleagues is a crucial protective factor in helping us to ensure that our observations are properly rounded, not distorted by our own prejudices, limitations or special professional interests. This process of second-order reflection on first impressions is a core aspect of good assessment practice. Experienced clinicians rely some of the time on the internalised self-supervisory capacities which can be built up over the years, but the complexity of the process of assessing a child or adolescent and their family is such that consultation with colleagues as we go along is a prime requirement.

The clinical setting needs to be as simple as possible and to be consistent. Meaning cannot be sensibly attributed to a child's differential response to a therapist between one session and another if the therapist has altered the setting. The same room, protection from interruption, pre-agreed times for the appointments, starting and stopping the sessions at the time arranged: these are the background factors which enable one to study the child's responses within a reasonably constant frame. This protected physical space and time supports the therapist in providing what is most needed – an uncluttered mental space, within which the emotional impact of the session can be contained.

Gathering enough clinical material to make a useful assessment can take variable amounts of time. Flexibility of approach is, of course, harder for clinicians – a more automatic standard model requires less case-by-case thinking – but its value in achieving real understanding of clinical problems and in safeguarding the primacy of patients being treated as complex individual human beings is great. Imaginative responsiveness to the needs of patients in the course of initial exploration is facilitated by a firm external structure, as described earlier, since it provides background security for the therapist. The encounter with what is *not known* is at the heart of an assessment, and this entails a good deal of anxiety for both patient and therapist (Bion, 1976) which the setting should make as tolerable as possible.

The technique described here depends on an understanding of the central role of transference in human relationships. The not-yet-familiar clinic and therapist and the emotional difficulties of the patient come together to elicit powerful unconscious patterns of communication. In addition to providing an opportunity for the child to express consciously what is on his mind, to tell his story as he sees it, there are other levels of meaning to be observed. The child's response to a receptive and observant listener can provide us with a picture of his fundamental ideas about the world, his inner convictions about himself and other people, some of which will be quite unfamiliar to his conscious mind. Does he expect to be understood or misunderstood, believed or distrusted, liked or disliked, worthy of attention or of no real interest?

The sessions will provide evidence of the child's unconscious feelings and beliefs but will also stir responses in the therapist. The therapist's feelings, nowadays often referred to a bit loosely as the 'countertransference', require careful thought, but if analysed in a rigorous way can often provide important additional data. Feelings which have their origins in the therapist's own personal world, conscious or unconscious, need to be put to one side. A patient whose problems feel too much like our own, or our children's, or whose history stirs echoes which trigger our anxieties, is likely to be a particular challenge. We need to be mindful of our own weaknesses. Therapeutic zeal, for example, can be based on self-idealisation of our professional capacities and can distort our clinical judgement. These are the sort of countertransference-based feelings which we need to become aware of and keep separate from our clinical judgement. There are, however, feelings stirred in us which do arise from the patient's impact on us. When quite unexpected feelings are registered by the therapist they can be an important clue to the patient's state of mind and need to be considered. The subtle power of projective identification as a form of communication (Bion, 1962a) underlies these phenomena.

If we find ourselves thinking that psychotherapy may be an appropriate recommendation, it is very useful to offer a taste of what this approach would entail for the patient and note its impact. Does this child feel helped or got at if one suggests links between one thing and another? Does he seem interested in his own mind, how he thinks and feels, or at a more primitive level, does he seem responsive to the idea that someone else – a therapist – would be interested in him? Does an interpretative comment lead to an opening out and deepening of communication, or a freezing, a defensive drying up or turning away? At the deepest level, it is the establishment of an openness to this sort of work that constitutes the 'informed consent' that we wish our young patients to give us. This is not primarily a matter of intellectual agreement, but consent to the emotional intimacy which will be the stuff of therapy. This may be more or less eager, but if one cannot see some evidence of desire for under-standing – though this may initially be the wish to be understood, which is not at all the same thing as understanding oneself (Steiner, 1993) – we are unlikely at this point to be able to make much thera-peutic impact.

The broad aims of our assessment will thus be to achieve the following:

- To establish whether there is someone who can reliably support the treatment of a child – parents or professionals with a role which can substitute for parents – or in the case of older adoles-cents, a more grown-up side of the adolescent's personality which can take responsibility to sustain ongoing treatment.
- To describe the child's state of mind, and to provide a preliminary formulation of the state of internal object relations, taking into account both developmental difficulties (deficits) and internal conflicts and defence systems.
- To describe the contribution of internal and external factors and to link with other workers to define priorities in the light of the overall balance (e.g. work with parents as a priority; levels of urgency in the child's need for individual treatment; work with school or social services required in parallel to or as preliminaries to psychotherapy).
- To clarify and make recommendations about action needed from other agencies to meet the mental health needs of the child and to have made proper use of the multidisciplinary team's resources: e.g. a psychiatric opinion where needed, an educational assess-ment where needed.
- To describe the patient's likely capacity to make use of psycho-analytic psychotherapy, to make a judgement about the appro-priateness of such intervention and to recommend the mode (individual, group or family), intensity and optimal timing of the treatment required.
- To establish a clear baseline of clinical description against which it will be possible to note changes which take place over time. The process of audit and of gathering data in such a way as to facilitate research possibilities needs to be built into assessment practice in

an ordinary way. Psychiatric classificatory systems, which empha-sise a different range of phenomena, have limited usefulness in clarifying the potential for psychotherapeutic treatment. Much work remains to be done to refine dynamically based clinical cat-egories and thus contribute to 'best practice'.

- To have offered the child/young person/family a therapeutic experience which provides containment of psychic pain and sus-tains hope, and which does not re-traumatise unwittingly through repetition of earlier environmental failure.
- To ensure that the time-frame of the assessment has been adequate to allow for a process of working through what is being proposed with child, parents and any other significant figures e.g. social worker. This will involve at least one meeting to review the pro-cess and outcome of the assessment sessions. In some cases more such meetings are required to punctuate a long and complex piece of work. Time is often required for the family (or the adolescent) to go away and think about what is being proposed before making a commitment. Decisions made too easily or hastily often mean that difficulties erupt in the course of therapy which are damag-ing to a child's well-being. Time devoted to gaining real consent is always worthwhile. The assessment process can be likened to setting in place the good foundations which enable buildings to have stability and durability.

The starting point in any individual case is bound to vary. For exam-ple, the assessment of an adolescent who may come to the clinic as a single member of a family, or perhaps feel very little sense of fam-ily connection at all, needs to be done in a way which is mindful of the child who grew into the person we meet at this point, even though the adolescent himself may feel very far from such a perspec-tive. Similarly, the troubles of children and adolescents can inform our understanding of their parents' conflicts and insecurities, though this might be a quite unfamiliar idea to parents who feel they are presenting their problematic child for help, not themselves. The intense flow of feeling between children and parents, which is often lifelong, is partially an expression of transferences within the family (Harris & Meltzer, 1986) and these are by no means uni-directional. Capacities for concern and caring which we associate with parental functioning can sometimes be observed in children towards their parents and siblings, while sometimes parental figures themselves may manifest little in the way of what a child might hope to find in those they depend on. The preconception (Bion, 1962b) of a responsive caring person, the 'good object' of psychoanalysis, sometimes seems to survive very damaging actual experiences, and conversely, the difficulty in benefiting from good care may be helpfully understood as a consequence of the domination of malign inner expectations (Henry, 1974).

Finally, it should be said that the opportunity to undertake initial exploratory work with a child can be a very special one. The freshness of the child's first communications makes assessment work a privilege and a source of extraordinary interest for the clinician. The anxiety of facing the unknown is balanced by the delight of discovery and the opportunity of a new beginning. A good assessment interview can be a crucial creative experience for a child in trouble.

5

FINDING A WAY TO THE
CHILD (1982)

I am going to describe some assessment work with the only child, a six-year-old boy, of a divorced mother.

The family had been referred to the clinic by their GP who was asking for psychotherapy for mother, which had been previously recommended at another clinic, and indicating that the child's state of mind and health gave considerable cause for concern.

Mrs. S. had consulted her GP about her persistent headaches and leg pains, and about Alex's hair, which was falling out. Hospital investigations suggested that all their symptoms were fundamentally psychosomatic and not organic. Some months later, mother again expressed worry about Alex, who was speaking of "wanting to die", saying that he would use a knife, and also sleepwalking. His mother felt he was disturbed by his frequent visits to his father – agreed access was three times weekly.

When this case was first considered, we thought it likely that both mother and son might need individual therapy. The degree of somatisation was worrying, but mother's persistent search for help was also striking. We felt concerned to provide a framework in our initial contact which could help her to distinguish between her personal needs and those of Alex – we had to devise an approach which took account both of her own difficulty and of her parental worry and active concern about Alex.

We decided to offer her an exploratory consultation with a social worker to sort out whether she wanted assessment for Alex, whether a treatment might be feasible practically, and to clarify the legal situation vis-a-vis care and control of the boy. A consultation took

DOI: 10.4324/9781003325543-8

place in which it was explained to her that a therapist could be available for her subsequent to an assessment of Alex, and that a decision would be taken jointly with her about what help would be appropriate for him. Our initial work was therefore designed to try to clarify whether there was available a parental framework of responsible concern which would provide a reliable setting for work with the child. Mrs. S. accepted this approach and kept to the appointments arranged, which involved a longish gap between exploration with her and assessment of Alex because of the summer holiday period.

I offered Mrs. S. two assessment sessions for Alex to be followed by a meeting between myself and her to discuss the implications of what I had observed. When I went to the waiting room to greet them, I met a very grubby looking, somewhat plump little boy, who made a tight and miserable first impression. Mother seemed warm and supportive towards him and he came with me without demur. In my room he went straight for the materials I had put out for him – drawing things, plasticine, small figures, animals and cars, scissors etc. – and without a glance at me or the room he began to play with them. I was not sure if he listened to my explanation about my role, the two meetings we would have, and so on. He took out a car and made it drive several times, head-on into the plastic bucket which held all the toys, giving me a feeling of brutal impact. He then took out the plasticine and seemed to consider making something, but rejected it in favour of the doll figures. An intricate non-stop game began, in which events succeeded each other at lightning speed. The original set-up was of two families, one composed of mother and a boy doll, the other of grandmother (called mother), big boy (actually the father doll), various smaller children (called babies), and miscellaneous other adults. The smaller and larger boys were fighting throughout, with murderous intent and great viciousness.

Most of my enquiries were ignored, but Alex did tell me that the anger of the smaller boy was because he was jealous of the babies in the other family – he had no babies in his house. The murderous attacks, so vividly enacted, led to continuous involvement of the police, the bigger 'boy' being taken off to prison, but never actually arriving and being held there, the smaller one when he was hurt being taken off by ambulance to hospital – he did not arrive either because the scene was changing too fast for any sequence to be completed. Alex half turned to me to explain: "He can't go to prison because he's under 21", and when the ambulance arrived he added: "They're taking him to hospital even though he's bad!" This was said in an expressionless tone of voice. I tried to interest him in the idea that this clinic where his Mum had brought him to see me might be a worrying place because he might not be sure whether it was a place for helping people who were hurt or ill or for punishing people who were bad. Alex shook his head, and said no, he didn't think so.

In the game, the membership of the family groups changed continuously, and the moral status of the combatants was volatile. Themes which reappeared were the smaller boy's protection of his mother and the intense rivalry between the two boys, which was often shown by one climbing up on top of the head and shoulders of the other, claiming superior strength and pressing, as if to push the victim down into the ground. The nature of the physical struggle was tremendously cruel, with particular attacks on each other's eyes, mouth, and genitals, and full of magical acrobatic feats.

I devoted my energies to trying to follow what was happening, and this Alex seemed to want me to get clear – when I would recap a sequence to express my understanding of it, he would correct me carefully if I had misunderstood him, and in his rather clumsy speech would pause momentarily to keep me on track. I tried to make contact with him by talking about the violence and cruelty and the rage of the doll figures, and about the confusion everyone seemed to be struggling with – who was in which family, who was good and who was bad, who was friend and who was enemy – but the game went on relentlessly and Alex showed no interest.

I found myself reviewing my own situation in the interview: I was witness to an interminable horror-story. Death was no end, since the protagonists were continually dying but immediately leaping to their feet and carrying on. I was struggling with an immensely confusing sequence of events in which no fixed point could be established – all relationships were changing constantly. The barrage of torture, pain, hatred, and fear was increasing, and no framework of meaning which could make sense of why any of this was happening could be grasped. A numb state of shock and a tense doom-laden expectation of more to come predominated.

I began to talk to Alex about how frightened and despairing all of these characters must feel and as I tried to put this idea into words, I felt a slight change in his emotional state. I could observe a lessening of his muscular tension, which had, up to this point, been holding him taut and motionless except for his hand movements, and he turned in his chair a little in my direction. The relentless pace of events in the game slowed down a bit. Feeling that I had established a small area of understanding between us, I asked about things he was afraid of. He turned around and looked at me, and halting the game told me about being frightened when Mummy goes out. He feels she will be kidnapped. At night he is afraid of burglars – they want to kill him and his Mummy with a knife.

They are under his bed. I asked if these were bad dreams he had and he agreed, but the borderline between the nightmare and the wide-awake phantasy of danger seemed minimal. While Alex was telling me this, he seemed to be feeling some anxiety for the first time – he took hold of the plasticine and twisted it around in his hands, not making anything, but having something to hold on to – but my main impression was of a child who had gone almost blank with fear. His face was expressionless, but it was as if too much had passed and nothing could any longer be transformed into communicable form. The dry facts about terror were all that was left. I felt it was important for me to go on talking to him, and to speak quietly and slowly, and to try to create a frame for the experiences of this session, so I talked about the clinic as a place where children could talk about fears and worries, his need for me to understand about how frightened he was, and explained that we would arrange with Mummy in the waiting room at the end of the session for him to come and see me again next week, when he and I could talk some more about this and think about what would help him. He nodded intently. I talked to him about his mind being completely full of the things he had been showing me, leaving no room for anything else, and at this point his face seemed to show a glimmer of sadness and I experienced him as extremely vulnerable. After he had packed the toys away, I found myself to my surprise asking if he would like to wash his hands – he was dreadfully grubby, and seemed to enjoy his perfunctory rinse and wipe, and I was left pondering the very concrete impact that his appeal for care had made on me.

When we returned upstairs to the waiting room he wanted to turn his back on me very quickly and get back to school. When his mother brought him for the second interview a week later, I noticed there was a man accompanying them; Alex made no reference to him although he is mother's co-habitee of some months' standing.

The session began in a very similar vein. The cruelty escalated, with overt torture seeming now to be the aim of each of the two boys – not just to be the winner but to inflict extremes of pain and humiliation on the other. The desperation of each contender to be on top was also intensified, the acrobatic feats attempted were of Superman proportions, and Alex spoke of both Superman and Spiderman when describing what was going on. The mother figure was now less protected from the violence, and got more and more involved on one side and the other.

A new theme emerged: Alex built a prison of plasticine where the three main figures were placed and detained by being dug deep – half buried, in fact – and he spoke of the huge weights on their feet and hands which were to prevent them escaping. When they did so, they were returned and the weights increased. This seemed a very vivid enactment of his experience of being deeply stuck in all these preoccupations and in despair about being able to free himself. The repetitious and doomed attempts to get free seemed an eloquent plea for an intervention which would allow some new element in, and betoken the possibility of change. For although the pell-mell activity continued, creating an illusion of speedy change and excitement, the overall impression grew of a quite deathly and timeless stasis, which would absorb whole lifetimes and beyond.

I began to talk again and said to Alex that I thought he needed to come to the clinic to see someone who would help him to think about all these frightening ideas that he felt stuck with. I explained that I would discuss this with Mummy, that I thought she wanted him to have this kind of help, and that I hoped we could then arrange for him to come regularly. I explained again that he would not be seeing me, but that I would find someone who could work with him here.

All this took some time to convey, and as he took it in, he stopped his game, took out a black pen, and began to draw. He drew a picture of White Land, which he connected with space and the moon.

This seemed to be a good place that he was going to travel to, but very speedily the paper began to fill with all kinds of elaborate weaponry to deal with the attackers who were expected. He talked quite easily to me about all this. I was interested both by the content of this picture, but even more so by the change in mode of communication – it seemed to me that when I had managed to create for him an idea of a clinic that was here to deal with his sort of worries, and that he experienced as real in so far as he felt me to be in touch with him, a fresh hope had kindled that there might be some good place that he could reach in his imagination. One might liken this to a baby waking up in a miserable persecuted frame of mind but nonetheless able to respond to the care offered by mother and to recognise her as something he was seeking. In Alex's situation, the care he requires seems particularly to be connected with being able to deal with a great deal of dirt felt as immensely powerful and blocking him off from anything more alive. He reminded me of the sort of baby who cannot possibly settle to feed or look around him until his dirty nappy has been dealt with. At the end of the second session, I was interested to note that he went to the basin in my room to wash, indicating his memory of the sequence of the earlier session, but initiating it himself.

In this case, the external frame for treatment of the child was in fact a solid one – despite grave personal difficulties for which mother was seeking help, she was able to be thoughtfully aware of her son's problems and was prepared to engage in treatment despite quite long journeys and father's opposition. She had some support in this from her boyfriend whom she brought with her to meet me and discuss Alex.

In the child's internal world, there was little evidence of a thinking frame which could help him to encompass his very complicated and confusing experiences. It had all been far too great a strain on an immature mind; in his real experiences his father invited him into a perverse collusion against mother, and his mother by her confused identification with his distress had been unable to provide any adult boundaries to protect him appropriately. However, in the assessment interviews, there was evidence that Alex could make use of a containing framework when I found a way to convey such a conception to him. I think this became a meaningful experience for him because I survived a degree of immersion in his nightmare world but emerged able to talk to him, so that he knew that I understood where he was.

Now I want to consider the experience I had with Alex in terms of my approach to the assessment of children for psychotherapy. The setting I offered was designed to make it possible for him to communicate with me about his inner world. This particular child's most urgent statement to me was not to be found in the content of his play and conversation but in the demonstration that the interviews provided of the monolithic character of his preoccupations. He was unable to respond to any ordinary enquiries about himself, what he liked, school, friends, and so on. The world in which he might be said to be living if one looked at it from outside was in fact being crucially shaped by the powerful phantasies of his internal world which occupied his entire mental space. The impoverishment of his capacity to make contact with reality was the result of an as-yet uncontained phantasy life. One detail of the play in the second session relates to this particularly – in the plasticine prison, huge lumps of plasticine were fashioned into weights on the prisoners' heads which also covered their eyes, so that they existed in a world of darkness which could not be penetrated, and they had no functional perceptual apparatus for seeing.

Talking with his mother amplified this picture – she described how he was viewed at school as being in a world of his own, how unable he was to learn despite his teachers' conviction of his intelligence. She also spoke of the nature of his play with other children – they had to play his games, which were always to do with death, and mother could describe how he successfully bullied his companions into the roles he designed for them. He was always the goody in these games, often with superhuman capacities, identified with one of the superheroes as he had shown me, since only characters like these had a chance against the forces of omnipotent destruction of which he was so fearful.

The assessment I made was intended both to inform me of this child's situation in terms of emotional development and capacity for experience and to give me some indication as to whether change might be facilitated by a clinical intervention. For this reason, the technique I use in assessing children has elements of the attitude I would adopt in an ongoing treatment setting, for I want to explore what use the child seems able to make of me and an unstructured interview. Whilst not interpreting any personal transference that I observe, I would want to test out the child's openness to linking comments, drawing together different aspects of what he shows me. I also find it important to keep a close eye on the emotional impact the child makes on me, and to think about the implications of this countertransference evidence in coming to conclusions about treatability. In other words, I am using the assessment process to review the possibility of change in a patient being facilitated by a therapeutic setting and relationship. So the concepts of change which inform psychoanalytic psychotherapy also permeate my initial contact with a child although there are many important differences too.

The sessions with Alex demonstrated a very rudimentary capacity to form a relationship. Most of the time, I felt myself not experienced as another person in the room with him at all. He seemed neither to feel he was in my room nor that the toys put out for him had been arranged by me. However, what took place did indicate to me that at a much more primitive level he was aware of a need to be listened to and kept in mind. He was able to elicit in me a sense of how to manage the situation for him in a way which would give him an idea that I could know about what filled his thoughts; in the way I talked to him, and by my attitude, I could convey to him that I had a capacity to think about him. He felt the superheroes were his only hope but he seemed able to perceive that a grown-up ally might be of some use.

6

WHAT FOLLOWS FAMILY BREAKDOWN?

Assessing children who have experienced deprivation, trauma, and multiple loss (1993)

Children may lose continuity of care within the family they entered at birth for a variety of reasons. In this chapter, the focus will be on children who have experienced severe losses. Such children are those whose families have been unable to provide an ongoing home and who have entered the system of child-care administered by the state. Either because of requests for help in taking care of a child from overwhelmed families or because of state intervention to remove a child from an abusive home, these children become the responsibility of social work agencies and are in residential homes or foster-placements, and some ultimately in adoptive homes. Within this group, the children referred for psychotherapeutic assessment are not usually those for whom there are hopes and plans for rehabilitation within the family of origin, but those for whom long-term alternative plans are being or have been made. They are the children who have not been helped enough by being offered alternative care, and whose psychological distress is evident either through their own visible unhappiness and difficulties in living, or through the disturbing effect they have on their carers and the wider world.

The task of assessment has several strands. It is useful to distinguish between the external and internal aspects of the overall situation. External factors include the feelings, wishes, anxieties and vulnerabilities of the adults responsible for the child's welfare at

DOI: 10.4324/9781003325543-9

home and at school, as well as the realistic options for ongoing care and possible treatment. Internal factors are those deriving from the nature of the child's internal world and its effect on his or her capacity for relationships, and for learning.

The assessment has to attend to whether intervention would be appropriate; to clarify who is looking for help and whether such help is available; to consider issues of timing; and to consider different forms of treatment and what problems could and could not be addressed through the varieties of possible therapies. These broader aspects of assessment involve exploration of the context and meaning of the referral to the professionals and other adults involved, and the nature and quality of the commitment of the parental framework around the referred child to ongoing specialist help. Alongside judgements on these matters is the accessibility of the child to psychotherapy, and the assessor's task of balancing the indications for and against individual psychoanalytic work with the child. The final task of the assessment process is the working through with child and responsible adults of the conclusions which emerge from the exploration undertaken. Perhaps it is misleading to use the term "final", since this needs to be the ongoing framework of all the encounters during the assessment: it has to be a process of dialogue, of two-way communication and sharing of understanding and of what is not yet understood, and a satisfactory outcome is one where all parties can accept that some shared thinking has taken place, and that the proposed intervention integrates the perspectives available.

There are technical problems and choices to be made in the course of such assessment work to which it will be useful to return after some discussion of clinical examples. Whereas it is necessary to have some models of how to structure assessment, I want to argue that models need to be maximally flexible, and are least useful when they prescribe how these tasks can be completed. The fundamental model I will be drawing on raises the following issues for investigation:

1   Who carries parental responsibility for the referred child? Can this be firmly located? This can be lost in the complex networks of, for example, foster parents, social worker, and school, and even more so in residential placements.
2   Who is experiencing psychic pain? Is it acknowledged?
3   Who is asking for help? A child has been referred, but it may not be the child who wants help.

4   Is there a recoverable narrative of the child's history? Such children often bring a history full of lacunae. How has this been negotiated thus far?
5   How much access can I get to underlying conflict and anxieties? How rigid are defences?
6   What is the response in the course of the assessment to emotional pain? Can it be tolerated if support is offered?
7   What indications can be gleaned from countertransference feelings? Do I feel motivated to help and if not, why not?

There is, however, one crucial point to take account of in approaching the work. The assessment has been requested because losses probably associated with other traumata have not been bearable and the intervention has to be designed to contain and not exacerbate any re-evocation of painful feelings related to loss. This is a difficult task. Children traumatised by losses which have overwhelmed their reflective capacities for understanding are extremely vulnerable to hurt. If they open up to a psychotherapist, the end of an assessment session may feel a cruel interruption or rejection. If there is likely to be a wait between assessment and a vacancy for ongoing therapy, they may feel abandoned in an exposed and inadequately protected mental state. If they have responded to repeated loss by resorting to more superficial relationships, they may rush into premature but shallow involvement and enthusiasm for the therapist. If frozen and guarded as a defence against hurt, they may seem inaccessible and be very vulnerable to despair about themselves if the hope they do not dare to espouse is not taken into account. These examples do not constitute an exhaustive list, but do emphasise the need for delicacy, clarity and courage: we are dealing with extreme psychological pain; there is scar tissue and poor healing of which we need to be aware.

One matter on which we can be reliable is what we ourselves offer. Whatever the sequence of interviews undertaken, it must always be clear what the next step is, and when it will take place. Loose ends are terrifying for children with experience of catastrophe and unpredictability. This means that if the assessment is being undertaken by someone who would not be able to offer ongoing therapy, this needs to be clarified at the outset, as it can otherwise be experienced as akin to seduction and betrayal. This often feels harsh to the therapist who has to face that s/he is making a limited offer to the patient, but we are protecting our own wish to be seen as benevolent at the expense of the patient if we do not make matters clear.

For psychotherapy to be viable, there has to be a clear locus of parental responsibility; otherwise confusion will ensue between therapist as a potential transference figure who can assist through engagement with the internal world of the child and therapist as a replacement parent. The pressure within a child who has lost parents to "find" them in the person of the therapist is enormous, and great care has to be exercised to prevent unreal hopes being aroused in the child, hopes for example that the therapist is the long-lost blood mother or hopes for a child waiting to be adopted that *this* is the person who will adopt him. Externally, this can be supported only if someone has made a real commitment to the parental task. This can be undertaken either by adoptive parents, or by a social worker in conjunction with parents or foster parents (or both), or by a statutory social worker in conjunction with residential social workers charged with the care of the child. Particular attention needs to be paid to ways in which, when there is a complex network of shared responsibility, there can be an enactment of diverse views between different people. Sometimes these splits in the professional network can mirror the extreme splits in the child's internal world, and when this is so they are particularly powerful. But they can also represent divergent ideological approaches to child-care, or inter- or intra-agency rivalry. Some of these themes are explored most usefully in Britton's chapter in *Psychotherapy with Severely Deprived Children* (Boston & Szur, 1983). Although the legal framework has changed recently, the fundamental model described by Britton remains pertinent. The child has to be someone's child, and to have a place in someone's mind.

I should like to contrast two assessments, the first in which there were functioning parents, in the sense defined earlier, and the second in which these were lacking. Each involves two children, half siblings. These assessments also draw attention to the difficulties and the importance of working closely with any other professionals involved in the case. Here, too, the dangers of destructive splitting between co-workers can be seen: psychoanalytically trained professionals are not immune to replacing thought by enactment! In my examples, effective co-operation within the Clinic took place in one case and not in the other.

Lorraine and David, aged 14 and 10, were referred by their social worker and prospective adoptive parents, with whom they were already living. There was a fairly detailed history available: the children had been removed from their unsupported mother's care aged five and one, together with another sister aged three, who had been badly hurt in an accident in the home when the children were left alone. This episode followed many previous occasions of neglect and abuse. The injured child was placed for adoption, following hospital treatment. The other two remained together, and had been in children's homes and in a long foster-placement which ended in their being very hurtfully rejected. A psychiatrist colleague in the Clinic had met with both social worker and adoptive parents to discuss the children's earlier lives, their current difficulties and the long-term care plans, which were for adoption to go ahead. Both children were in some difficulties at school and were not easy to live with, and the parents hoped that therapy might help them to make better use of the family life they were committed to offering.

I decided to begin by seeing both children together, since the one constant factor in their turbulent lives had been their living together. I wanted to observe the nature of their involvement with each other, and then planned to see them individually on a later occasion.

I had not by any means anticipated the tumultuous session that took place. David was small for his age, fair-haired, neat, a live-wire child; Lorraine, by contrast, was big, gawky, dark and looked younger than her years. They had been looking at a "baby" book in the waiting room, with Lorraine sitting in a baby chair, and were joking about who was the baby. David made an immediate impact, anxious about what to do with the drink he had been given from the vending machine and passionately demanding to go down to my room in the lift. I felt it was urgently necessary to get a firm grip and said that we would walk down but could come up by lift at the end.

I had put out a selection of small toys on a low table in the middle of my room, and drawing materials on the desk by the window. David headed for the toys but then saw that Lorraine had sat down, so did likewise. I spoke briefly about this being an opportunity for me to get to know them, and indicated that the toys and drawing things were for them to use. Their eyes met and a prolonged giggle broke out. David's giggle was violent and loud, and gave the impression of his progressively working himself up to a high. There were noisy mutual accusations: "You're making me laugh". As the giggling persisted, I spoke about the pleasure of having a good giggle together, probably much nicer than wondering about me whom they did not know or wondering what they should do here. Infectious outbursts continued apace so I talked about their embarrassment, and after a while commented on the theme of their noisy laughter filling up the room and leaving no empty space. This remark made contact, and they began to investigate the toys. The chaos and noise was tremendous, however, and rivalry dominated everything. They squabbled, snatched and chattered abusively. David was full of dirty talk and kept up a torrent of verbal abuse of Lorraine and she retaliated by hitting his head.

Surveying the scene, I felt I had two very wild toddlers in the room, in overgrown bodies. I talked determinedly about my wanting them to tell me about themselves, and David then launched into the story of the injury sustained by the third sibling. Mother was silly, he said, she had gone out and left them alone. During this narrative, the noise and perpetual distraction continued, but I managed to get reasonably clear their picture of what had happened and to find out about current contact with this sister. I said something about how horrible and frightening this must have been, to which they agreed, but any attempt to get them to go on with the story of what happened next met with a blank wall and further waves of excitement and noise.

The children decided to draw. This also became an argument, each wanting the other's pencil which seemed sharper than their own, and this despite the presence of a sharpener. David was very restless, and interfered with Lorraine who drew slowly and carefully, and with enjoyment. David drew a witch with a spider coming out of her nose saying "kill me". I asked to whom was she saying it and he said "to Lorraine", pushing the picture at her. "What would happen?" I asked: "she'd be frightened", he replied. He then drew a giraffe with measles, "a special disease that only farts get", he announced. Then he scribbled a horse, in imitation of Lorraine's carefully drawn horse. Lorraine had drawn two horses, the first a show-jumper "whose head was too big", she said, the second a patchwork horse "tired after a long ride". She did not know whether its head was down because it was tired or because it was eating, but then added grass and said the horse was like a lawn-mower. She talked about going horse-riding herself. Her arm was recently broken as the result of a fall, and she showed me her distorted arm. She handed both pictures to me and said, "They're for you". She was quiet now, and basking in my attention. This hopeful turning towards me had a most touching quality.

92

Meanwhile David went to play with the bricks. I sat between the children trying to watch and listen in both directions. David's play had two phases. First, there was a lengthy game of building shaky towers, bulldozing them down with cars or simply using his hands to sweep them to pieces. The pleasure seemed to be in the moment of smashing it all up. He began to talk about the leaning tower of Pisa and why it leaned, and both children got involved in speculations about this – what would happen if it fell? Gradually, David's manic delight in the crashes faded and he began to get frustrated and a bit miserable that he could not build higher.

I now felt I could formulate an anxiety they both shared and had expressed in their own ways and I spoke about their both feeling there was a problem about things not balancing well – Lorraine's horse's head was too big, David's towers got top-heavy. Was something a bit too much to manage? I was thinking of an image of a head/mind that could not contain something so burdensome. Of course they had shown me this problem in a direct way, in that the question I myself had been faced with was whether I could manage them. I had certainly been oppressed by thoughts of how much the racket they were making would be disturbing nearby colleagues and other patients. After this intervention, David's building techniques improved, and he enjoyed his success hugely. I thought that I had perhaps contained his anxiety adequately through this interpretation. He also began to display what struck me as a very lively intelligence, for his quick wit was now directed not at tormenting Lorraine but at observing all the different kinds of brick and working out variations on how they could be fitted together.

Lorraine had been talking about Easter holiday plans, rather excited and muddled at the idea of visiting adoptive mother's mother, and also about the operation she would have soon to insert grommets in her ears. She explained all this very well, about the liquid behind her ears, her permanent cold and her hope that when her nose had been cauterised she would be free of all the thick catarrh. She was in fact very obviously troubled by this symptom. I wondered in my own mind about thoughts she might have about the Clinic – might there be something done for her here too, which would make her feel better? She moved over to the table where David was working and played briefly with the little dolls and animals. There was another episode of snatching each other's things, but then David concentrated on a particularly elaborate building and both children became involved in this. A much quieter tension now held the air as I wondered whether this building too would be demolished. In fact the vehicles were driven round at a dangerous pace with accompanying screeches of brakes etc., but with dramatic swerves, like cars on a race track avoiding skids, and they would be brought to a halt inches from catastrophe. While this was proceeding both children were at the small table engaged in the same game. I had noticed the shape of the building and when they asked me what I thought it was called I replied straightforwardly that it had made me think of Buckingham Palace. David confirmed with delight that I had guessed correctly. I was sure that this game held a shared meaning for them and I surmised that this concerned the depth of their preoccupation with the issue of whether this "palace", which I felt represented the admired and overwhelming material and emotional riches of their new home, was strongly enough built to survive the impact of their destructiveness. Also in question was whether their feelings of wonder and gratitude at what they were being offered would be able to contain their powerful impulses to attack and spoil, to test to destruction.

I was much impressed in this session by the joint defences these two had constructed – excitement powered by hilarity and obscenity held anxiety at bay quite effectively, and their mutual clinging relieved potential loneliness and the terror of facing so many worries about themselves and their future. David had a powerful personality and a sharp intelligence, but despite the array of manic defences I thought it had been possible to reach through to make contact with his vulnerability quite quickly. Lorraine seemed less secure, anxious to find things to hang on to.

I decided next to see each child separately, and I will describe briefly the striking contrast these sessions presented.

Lorraine began uncertainly, and I spoke about the discomfort of David not being there. After a brief conversation recalling the joint session – "those bricks!" she giggled – she began to draw. She sketched a complicated chart of the universe, earth, sky, the planets etc., and got lost in trying to remember the names of the planets. Setting this aside, she drew an Easter picture which she said came out the wrong way round: "I always do that", she added. Next she made an Easter card. I talked to her about the chart being an attempt to show me a picture of the world she felt she lived in, both the outside world and the world inside her, her memories, the past and the present, her first family and now her new family. She was showing me how many gaps there are – it doesn't quite make sense to her. I reminded her of the long gap of years in the story of their lives as they had told it to me. She then drew my attention to a mistake she made, writing "4" instead of "E", which I took as a possible entrée to more talk about the new family of four. However, Lorraine did not really listen to me and the amazing thing was that despite the peace and calm of the session, in contrast to the tumult of the earlier one, I was now feeling concerned at the degree of her deafness – she had been able to "hear" far more in all that noise than she could now!

She involved me in a companionable game with the animals in which I was to make a zoo for the wild ones while she made a farm for the domestic animals. We could be quite cosy together on the basis of ignoring any difficulties and any painful feelings and playing a little girl game together. I felt under a lot of pressure to be pleased by the gift of pictures and good wishes for Easter, to accept her surface friendliness and not to challenge her underlying boundary-lessness. This was evident as she packed up when she said "till next time". This seemed to negate all the work I had put into explaining that I would be seeing her just this once to help me think with her parents about whether coming to the Clinic regularly to see someone else might help her. I was left with considerable anxiety: her limited intelligence and somewhat shallow capacity for attachment seemed manifest, but I also had evidence that a great deal of blocking-out was going on which would make it difficult to make contact with the troubled child within. She did not *feel* anxious and she certainly did not want to have to, at this point.

David on his own, by contrast, was openly worried and talked about how nervous he was without Lorraine. "It was better when she was here" he said. He spoke in a quiet confiding voice, and I felt he was afraid to hear and feel his own anxiety so clearly. He went back to the bricks, and tower-building, and more crashes caused by the cars. The destructive car was driven by Lorraine, he announced, and he, David, was driving the dump-truck and trying to intervene and deal with Lorraine's attacks. He was quite clear that he was the good one and she the bad one. I wondered about some feelings of his own about smashing things up which he had showed me last time. He then constructed an elaborate building. Again Lorraine's vehicles approached dangerously, and David with his ally Superman worked at protecting it. I tried to link this with his worries about things falling to pieces in his life more than once – and referred to the missing years of their narrative. "It's too private", he said. "I can't talk about it". His voice had become absolutely tiny and I was thus made aware of how small and frail he felt in relation to really overwhelming worries about the destructive potential within himself and Lorraine.

The game changed to going into space, to search for a lost star. He spoke of a mystery. "When it comes to earth, something will come to life again". When I picked up his questions about himself, his own story, what had got lost, he became quite anxious – when will he come here again? How long is he going to stay? I talked about the possibility of ongoing work at the Clinic, and he said "With Lorraine would be better" and then wanted to leave early to get home in time for Tarzan on TV. I tried to encourage him to stay and he produced a stream of drawings of TV heroes. "They help people" he said, as he hummed the theme tunes, feeling safe again with his omnipotent protectors close at hand. On the back he drew a steam train with lots of coal and smoke, and at this unconscious allusion to the anal preoccupations more evident in the earlier session he became really anxious to leave.

These sessions provide abundant material relevant to the questions raised in my model of assessment. Both children had affected me powerfully with a wish to help them, though I knew that I could not undertake the ongoing therapy personally. The evocative, even haunting quality of their play and verbal communications lodged in my mind. I would understand this as a communication received by me in the countertransference of their wish to be helped, as well as of their anxieties about themselves. In the sessions, much of the impact on me was registered fleetingly, and it was in the subsequent reflection on the interaction that some of the unconscious aspects of the countertransference could be brought to mind, and made use of in my understanding. This mulling over of the experience of the session is a fundamental part of the assessment process. Allowing time to think over what has happened, to let it gather meaning gradually, is necessary for the conscious and unconscious material to be integrated in the mind. Premature formulations need to be avoided, and the structure of the assessment appointments offered can facilitate access to the process of reverie (Bion, 1962a).

I had evidence of the extent to which the children's actual capacities were being crippled by maladaptive defences, predominantly manic hyperactivity, with unmodified splitting and projection. I had also learnt something of the pressure of anxiety about strength and survival in the face of impulsive destructiveness with which both the children and their adoptive parents were likely to be faced. My experience of being together with the two children in a room for one hour gave me a vivid glimpse of a clash of cultures: the two formed a sort of little gang (Waddell, 1998) which parental figures might find it very difficult to penetrate. The level of anxiety and frustration this might engender in adults trying to find their feet as parents of their children was not hard to imagine.

Becoming a family, in the sense of the children being able to trust the parents to respond to their more infantile dependent needs and help them to separate their own individual personalities gradually from the enmeshment I could observe was going to be a tough challenge.

What therapeutic approach was indicated? Despite the difficulty of fighting through the confusion and speed of events in the joint session, I thought I had in fact made more contact with the children's anxieties when I saw them together. They seemed to feel safe enough, when protected by their well-rehearsed repertoire of joint defensive manoeuvres to listen to me from time to time. In the individual sessions, despite excellent evidence for interpretive linking, I had encountered Lorraine's tendency to block, a sort of deafness, and defensive quasi-stupidity, and David's very easily unbearable degree of anxiety. Some disentangling of their mutual defensive system seemed a pre-requisite for useful individual psychotherapy to be possible.

The idea that a therapist could paradoxically have more space to engage the children in thinking in joint sessions matched an important external factor. Over the next year, the children's placement would be facing the strain of being tested for durability, and the legal processes of adoption would add to this stress. I thought it could be very helpful for the children to have a place to express their feelings about this shared life-crisis, and that this would be protective of the placement. Individual work could well follow at a later date.

Now, by contrast, here is a case example where children are being fought over by professionals, and where parental responsibility is thus not being exercised. The setting of this work was varied, involving both formal clinic appointments and visits to foster-homes, and such flexibility of approach can make an important difference in cases where the conflicts have become embedded in hostile professional staking-out of positions. The assessment issues in the case of Peter and Dan included at different times:

1 With whom should they live?
2 Should they be together?
3 Is psychotherapy needed?
4 How can social services be helped to make an effective plan for these two boys?

Dan is the younger of two brothers of mixed race. Mother, who had herself been brought up in care, in a succession of children's homes, received little support from Father with the children, either emotional or financial. Social services, who had continued to function as a surrogate family for her after she formally left their care, saw much of the two babies from the start, and worries abounded, as she seemed unable to cope, and there were repeated episodes of the children being exposed to physical risk. This culminated in the babies being taken into care and placed with a foster mother when Dan was five months and Peter fifteen months. At that time I had been involved in visiting them in their foster home as part of making a contribution to social services' deliberations about their future.

The bit of the story I want to focus on begins when Dan was about three. By this time, Peter had been placed in a residential therapeutic community and Dan was causing his social worker and foster mother much anxiety. Both boys had become sexually precocious and there was suspicion of sexual abuse during one of their foster placements, although a formal Child Sexual Abuse investigation had proved unproductive.

I was asked to assess Dan, to advise about what long-term placement should be sought and what treatment might be needed, and initially saw him twice in the Clinic. In those sessions I was worried about the nature of the present placement, as foster mother seemed so detached from Dan, who was an engaging, lively little boy. But I was impressed by the evidence of Dan's capacity to make a relationship with me within this brief contact, which developed from a too-quick willingness to attach himself to me to something more substantial. This is what happened.

Dan came with me easily. He had been playing on the wooden train in the waiting room, but accepted my hand and came happily, as if quite interested. He went straight to the toys I had put out for him and began to look through them while I explained about his coming to see me twice, and my wanting to get to know what sort of boy he was. He took out the bundle of pens, held together by an elastic band. He began to take the tops off, then removed the band so that they scattered on table and floor. After looking at all the colours, he seemed to want to put them together again, and was quite efficient at collecting the bits from the floor and matching them up. One he could not manage as it had come to pieces more radically and he gave it to me, indicating that I was to sort it out. All this while he was not speaking at all, although I described his activities to him and he seemed perfectly at ease. After a brief glance at the little bricks and the toys, and around the room, he settled on the floor by my feet and began to take out the little doll figures and examine them. He announced, (his first words), "This is you", as he took out the mother doll figure, looking at me. The dolls held his attention only briefly, being each held and then laid aside, and he then turned to the animals.

Picking up the largest animal, the rhinoceros, he said "Bogey-man", as if it were the animal's name. Then he briefly fingered each animal, quite often announcing that it was a bogeyman, as if making no discrimination at all between different animals. The only one to which he gave its correct name was the dog.

Hearing a noise outside he climbed up onto my desk, by the window, and looked out. He did not appear to expect me to object. After looking out at some road works, he became fascinated by the anglepoise desk lamp which he manipulated with careful curiosity. I was not clear what he thought it was. I remained very close by as he sat on the desk and investigated this, and I talked about what he was doing. He noticed that it was rather a bashed-up object, and drew attention to the bent bits, and tried to turn it on – it did not work at the moment, I explained to him. He fingered the bulb with interest and allowed me to prevent him doing anything dangerous. He then asked for a drink.

We went to the sink and got a beaker of water. He drank some and carried the rest carefully over to the desk and used it to wash the lamp, smoothing on water with his fingers and rubbing it over the dusty metal surface. With great devotion, he tried to get the lamp into better order.

While up on the desk, he was, at one point, distracted by the telephone which he wanted to be allowed to play with. I had to be very alert to make sure that his activities were safe – not too close to the window, not breaking the lamp bulb, etc. – and that he respected my limits, which meant not playing with the telephone or putting water on my papers. I found that he was quite containable with close attention. I talked to him about his worry about things that are broken or dirty and his wanting to show me how much he would like to mend things, and what a lot of hard work it took.

When the lamp work seemed done to his satisfaction, he climbed down. Kneeling at the table, he drew a few quick shapes and scribbles in different colours, but did not respond to my asking what he was drawing. The tall cupboard in the corner of the room attracted his attention. He went to it, saying "bogeyman". I wondered aloud if he was frightened about a bogeyman who could hide in cupboards. He pushed the door to, and kicked it a bit. Then he went to the sink, getting me to help by moving a chair so that he could reach, and he played at length with the water, pouring water collected in one cup into another. He accepted my limiting the flow of water, and played like a toddler at a kitchen sink with great contentment. He allowed me to help him get dry when it was time to leave.

For the second session he arrived very late, so we had only half the planned time. Dan was looking at a book in the waiting room. Mrs M, his foster carer, apologised for the lateness. I suggested he could bring the book with him if he liked, as he seemed reluctant to put it down, and I thought he might be feeling rushed as he had no time to get to feel at home in the waiting room. He knew the way to my room very precisely, leading the way at speed. Going straight to the toys, he examined the cow, looking at the udders and then at me. Next he picked up and correctly named the tiger and several more animals. He examined the crocodile. As he picked out toys, he put them to his mouth, giving little bites. Then more deliberately he picked up the cow, hit it and threw it back hard into the toy-bucket. Next he made the female dolls and animals fight each other.

He then tidied up the toys carefully and went to the desk, and briefly resumed similar play to last time with the lamp and the phone. "What's that?" he said, pointing to a bottle of ink. He accepted my removing this and seemed to want to put the desk in order. This led to the discovery of a small drawer containing office items which he examined closely. I talked about his interest in everything here, wanting to get it all sorted out. He then returned to the little table and began to draw. He told me his picture was "you", and then correctly named most of the colours of the pens he was using. Finding a slightly torn piece of paper, he said "who did that?" and asked for Sellotape to mend it, and later for the rubber he had used the week before which he had obviously remembered. He made various remarks about the rubber, as if to take possession of it for himself.

Then he played at the sink, interested in the plug and chain which had become detached. "Who broke it?" he asked, trying for a while to reconnect the two bits, and then, when he could not manage it, settling for playing with the water.

He returned to the corner cupboard, first looking at the drawers in the chest next to it, and trying to open them all. Then he spoke again of the bogeyman and seeing the cupboard lock tried to find a key which would enable him to lock it up firmly. I talked about his wanting the bogeyman to be put away, locked up, not to be able to interfere with what Dan wanted to do here or to frighten him.

When it was time to finish, he did a very thorough clean-up of all the many objects he had used, but left one small toy, a naked baby-doll, lying on the carpet, apparently unnoticed.

Discussion

The development in Dan observable in this second session was remarkable. He was much more able to use language, to make discriminations and to explore questions. He gave many signs of recall of the previous week's session.

Dan gave abundant evidence of an interest in, and capacity for, a relationship with a mother figure; he showed anxieties about damage but also some hope that repair was possible. I saw him as a child who could make good use of a suitable long-term family placement, and wrote a report on these lines, also suggesting that individual therapy could be considered once a family placement had been made, as it would support his capacity to make use of family life.

Six months later, I learnt that no action had been taken about permanent placement, that there had been a change of social worker, and of foster home, and that the new social worker felt that my comments were not in tune with the new foster mother's complaints about Dan's worrying sexualised state and his destructiveness. The social worker felt a re-assessment was needed, as he believed a period of time in a therapeutic community was needed by Dan. He was also much preoccupied by concerns about the child's racial identity and the constraints this placed on appropriate placement. I suggested that I visit Dan in his foster home and this proposal was accepted.

I arranged by telephone with Mrs P, the new foster mother, to visit one afternoon. She was a bit suspicious on the phone, but quite welcoming when I arrived. Three small children were playing in the living room area and she seemed pleased when I declined going into the "posh" room and suggested we stay where the children were. I introduced myself to her teenage son for whom she was cooking a late lunch, and sat on the sofa. Both Dan (now three and a half), and the two-and-a-half-year-old foster girl who was sharing this home immediately wanted my full attention and to sit on my lap. I said hello to each child individually. There was also a younger boy, about two, who Mrs P child-minds. Mrs P is of West Indian origin; Dan looks white, despite his mixed race background; and the other two children are black. The atmosphere in the house was easy-going. The son came and went, another friend visited, later Mrs P's nine-year-old daughter returned from school with a friend. There was a feeling of "open house", with all the older children and adults being friendly to the group of little children.

For the first quarter of an hour I was kept busy looking at a "book" (a shopping catalogue), brought to me by Dan. I talked to him about the times he came to see me at the Clinic, and my now coming to see him at his house. He was extremely friendly, as was Cheryl, the foster sister, in an overtly competitive way. She tried to get into my lap and exclude the others. The little one was more cautious, wanting to join in and imitating the other children, but less throwing himself at me. He sat by me, and I protected the possibility of all three seeing the book. Dan found it easier to share than Cheryl. He turned the pages and liked to look at the toy section – he was especially interested in a toy desk, and also in watches and clocks. Dan's language was clear. Cheryl copied his phrases frequently.

The children were entertained for a long time by our conversation about the book.

Dan mentioned Angela, who used to look after him sometimes, and several times spoke of "my brother". "My brother in Kent". He initiated conversation with Mrs P about Peter – "When did we go and see him? When can we go?" Mrs P said after Christmas, and at another time promised he could ring Peter up on Christmas Day to wish him Happy Christmas. She came and sat near after a while, when her cooking was done. When Dan asked for the bucket of

Lego, she took it off the fridge and gave some Lego to each child to play with. Dan got really involved in building a train "to go to Kent", he said. He had one play-person boy who he put on top of the train. He was skilful with the Lego pieces and had a good eye for what would fit where.

Mrs P went to fetch her daughter from school after a while and left the children in my care (!). They hardly seemed to notice her departure, but then became even more excited when she was out and kept me busy.

Later Mrs P asked if I had been told about Dan's "problem", and we moved to the other room. She described Dan's sexual play with Cheryl. Twice she had found him "attempting intercourse". Mrs P was clearly shocked by Dan's erection and very anxious to protect Cheryl. She felt that the children could not be left alone. She was worried that Cheryl would be seen as abused or become vulnerable to abuse. She also complained of episodes of wanton destructiveness – throwing things out of the window, for example a ring, and breaking things of particular value to other people in the house (for example, the TV, cassette player, etc.). Mrs P saw Dan as having a very affectionate, nice side, but suddenly on occasion becoming destructive. She did not think this behaviour could be sensed in advance.

In the latter part of this talk, Dan and Cheryl came into the room and played quite calmly, delighted by the Christmas tree and lights.

When I prepared to leave Dan expressed his crossness quite openly, hitting me, and then turning his back on me. Mrs P had stressed his appealing qualities, his lovability, and I too was struck by this.

I felt it made an impact on Dan when I tried to explain who I was and why we were together. I didn't imagine that he remembered me from my earlier contact when he was ten months old, although he was very recognisable to me as the same child, but I did think he was able to link up the earlier Clinic visits and my appearance in his home. I think he knew that it was relevant to tell me about his intense preoccupation with getting to see his brother. My awareness of the multiple changes and losses of his life up to this point was the background to his telling me so clearly who he felt he belonged with. (Mother, father, brother, two previous foster mothers and numerous foster siblings, and his first social worker had all disappeared, and all in fact in circumstances that must have been upsetting, if not worse).

The difficult behaviour Mrs P reported makes a lot of sense if one looks at it as potentially a communication about Dan's feelings – it was so striking to hear that this frequently thrown-away little boy was trying to find a way to draw attention to his feelings of being lost and thrown out. His destructiveness towards objects that other people particularly cared about seemed to me similarly poignant; his desperate wish to be precious to someone, to be held onto, was matched by jealous rage at what he perceived as favoured rivals. I suspected that his sexual approaches to Cheryl were to be understood as his inappropriate attempt to get close to her, to use sexual excitement as a glue to attach her to him, and as a manic denial of the many sad aspects of his life. The abandoning parents are so often experienced in the child's mind as having chosen excitement with each other in preference to caring for the children and we can often observe images of internal sexualised parents with whom the child identifies.

The concept of containment (Sorensen, 1997) provides a way of thinking about this boy's experience. The episode which had precipitated the children's reception into care had been when Dan, aged four and a half months, was left on top of a washing machine in the care of Peter. Such lack of safety and containment, either physical or mental, was unfortunately replicated by his experience in care in many ways. He was perpetually fought over by contending powers. I had, for example, been to one case conference where it was being proposed that he be given a day nursery place at the age ten months because his first foster mother was deemed to be inadequately stimulating, not providing the right educational toys. This was at a point when he was very much settled with her, and where his sense of belonging with her (in her arms, on her lap, in her kitchen) was palpable. The respect that needed to be given to the achievement of this relationship between Dan and foster mother was fearfully undermined by such interventions, in my view.

The lack of containment of Dan's not being able to rely on some boundaries of safety and common sense being maintained for him, played a big part in the pressures he would then place on each succeeding carer: the question remained open whether anyone would hang to him, whether he was going to belong to anyone. With such huge life issues at stake, it is sometimes hard to take seriously the helpfulness of even a small piece of work where some basic structure can be established and protected, but I think his use of me is a good demonstration that it is worthwhile to struggle with this. I had repeated doses of what Dan must have felt in my long contact with social services over this case. I never received acknowledgements of my written reports, I was frequently not sent minutes of case conferences, or my contributions would be omitted. In fact I only found out the outcome of the report I had written for social services on the basis of my home visit when I opened my newspaper one day some months later to see a large picture of the boys, part of an advertisement seeking a family for the two brothers.

Now, it is worth asking what factors make it so hard for professionals working under pressure to maintain what they would probably consciously accept as good practice – no-one thinks it is good for small children to spend the first three years of life in a succession of short-term placements, but it happens none the less. One of the ideas that helps in understanding this is the emotional effect on workers of their own response to their cases. The countertransference has diverse elements which can usually be distinguished. Firstly, there is the worker's own partly unconscious emotionality, which can be stirred up by the nature of the work. The personal resonance of feelings of loss, abandonment, damage, neglect and hope, repair, reconciliation can interfere with our judgement, because we can feel we are involved in our own life problems rather than those of the children we are responsible for. For example, I think that Dan and Pete's first social worker, who left the field altogether in a state of poor health and burn-out, had struggled without success to differentiate her feelings for these children from her feelings about her current situation in a collapsed inner London social services department. Cuts, reorganisation, changing policy guidelines, closure of local social services offices, all replicated too closely the issues within the case. Her helpless sense of being abused, sometimes over-ruled and sometimes left unsupported to bear the uncertainty and anxiety about her own and the children's future left her no mental space to think about them. Her professional identity was assaulted beyond the point of recovery. We know that the helping professions attract many who feel a personal identification with those they are trying to help and this involves a risk to the professional which needs to be minimised by supportive structures of professional practice and supervision.

In contrast, there is the element in the countertransference response which picks up and registers in feeling some of the significant

105

elements in the child's communications. Thought of in this light, our capacity for unconscious perception is a precious resource, if we can train ourselves to ponder on the curious details of the feelings stirred in us by our patients. The hurt and outrage which Dan's foster mother felt about his hurling out of valuable objects and his destructive mucking about with the communication systems within the house was such a revealing part of the story – he was forcing her to stand for him the anxiety of not being valued, of links and communication being broken, and to know within herself how hurt and furious he was about the way in which his life had been repeatedly disrupted. He could only express himself in action, partly because no-one was talking to him much about himself.

The danger is that our actions may be driven not by thought but by such powerful unconscious identifications. Mrs P had to work hard at times not to be provoked into yet another re-enactment of Dan's inner drama of his unacceptability and consequent rejection. I had to work hard not to explode with irritation as the social services' conflict about this family was enacted via yet another rival referral to an alternative expert agency. This process of splitting also took place *within* the Clinic – at the point when I was embarking on my assessment of Dan, a separate approach was made to a colleague with a specialist interest in Child Sexual Abuse disclosure work to do video interviews with both brothers for the police. I was not informed by the social worker or by my Clinic team colleagues of this until the work was already under way! It was hardly surprising that nothing of value could be clarified in the video interview since both the foster mother and the two boys probably experienced the Clinic as becoming incomprehensible – where was I, my room, my toys? Why had everything changed?

Our susceptibility to not being in control of ourselves rationally in the best interests of children in our care cannot be removed. Instead it has to be acknowledged, taken seriously and systematically considered. When we discover we are not in control of all our actions, let alone our emotions, it is an uncomfortable realisation. But perhaps this truth can also help us to understand better the emotions of children who feel that their lives are predominantly not under their control, so patently the case for children in care. They have difficulty in managing their own impulses and feeling states, and the ordinary system of care and control (and those two concepts need to be intrinsically linked if the control is to be of a helpful sort) has broken down. There are illusory ways of gaining control of things, often through violence or perversity, but these are terribly self-destructive.

An adopted child I am currently working with has been showing me in play with water and bubbles that an element of feeling one is making one's own world is part of becoming more humanly related. Babies initiate their own birth, to an extent which has only recently been realised, and this physiological fact is true of psychological life too. Powerlessness to influence one's fate is catastrophic of self. Illusory power, so characteristic of delinquent character structures, is insubstantial. Being able to have an effect on somebody is the beginning of relatedness, but being able to overwhelm people destroys relationships.

My assessment of Dan highlighted different issues requiring attention. Dan's own need continued to be primarily for a long-term family placement together with his brother. More frequent and reliable contact with his brother was an urgent immediate concern. The possibility of psychotherapy for him at a later date could also be noted but might not prove necessary. The social worker's anxieties about ethnic identity could be approached through an appreciation of what he himself as a black professional could offer these boys. The anxiety shared by social worker and foster mother about sexual acting-out and destructive behaviour could be addressed by giving meaning to Dan's behaviour and alerting them to the immensely painful losses which this little boy had sustained and the way in which he was trying to deal with these. This case is one in which the request for individual assessment (with the implication of individual psychopathology as the focus) needs a response taking the child's whole circumstances into account, identifying projections into the child and offering containment for the child's unheard communications. The task is to connect up the needs of the child with the potential responsiveness of the responsible adults.

Now I should like to discuss briefly the range of options I have in mind during assessment for psychotherapy. It may be appropriate to recommend individual therapy on either an intensive or once-weekly basis. For some very deprived children, once-a-week work has proved to be an optimal intervention, because it provides a bearable rhythm of exposure to intense emotions. It may also be all that is practicable either because of limited resources or because of the demands that bringing a child for regular treatment makes on the substitute family. As indicated in my first case example, joint work with siblings is also to be considered. If available, joining a children's psychotherapy group can be very helpful for some patients, particularly very persecuted and very inhibited children who can use the other members of the group to contain and express parts of their personalities with which they are unfamiliar. If the assessment reveals problems that are located more outside than inside the child, family therapy, work with the parents or consultation to the wider network may be indicated, at least as the initial step.

Because therapy with severely deprived children makes particular demands on the therapist, there are also linking factors with respect to choice of therapist. The degree of psychic pain and confusion to be faced is such that inexperienced therapists need a great deal of supervision and support to treat such cases. Containing the projected despair is a very taxing process and when a child's hopelessness gets entwined with a therapist's lack of confidence, it is difficult to make progress. But even very experienced therapists are likely to need access to professional support, as the children's terrors about their viability in life impinge very deeply. Some of them are likely to be physically violent at times during sessions, and this makes a Clinic setting very much more suitable than private practice, since it provides a sense of limits and safety which both child and therapist may need. Work with the substitute family, social worker, etc. is an absolutely essential adjunct to therapy with these children, and is best undertaken by a Clinic colleague with a commitment to protecting the structure of the child's psychotherapy. This is bound to be battered in the course of working through the child's doubts and suspicions. The final but immensely important point to be made is that treatment of this group of patients is a long-term commitment; they are more vulnerable than other children to anxieties about loss and change, and should be spared changes of therapist or disruption in their treatment if at all possible.

Despite all these cautionary reflections, my experience in assessing severely deprived children has often been particularly rewarding. The child psychotherapist is equipped to offer something which many of them have lacked an experience of in their early development and to which astonishingly many of them remain able to respond. It is a privilege to observe the eloquence in word or deed with which the opportunity to be understood is embraced. The theoretical developments in psychoanalysis which have made it possible for us to begin to understand traumatised and neglected children have opened our eyes and ears not only to evidence of pain but also to the potential for survival and recovery.

7

ASSESSING CHILDREN AND FAMILIES

Developments in a paradigm (1995)

In this paper I trace the history of changing understandings of what we mean by assessment and how we go about it. When I first arrived at the Tavistock to train as a child psychotherapist in 1968, assessments were undertaken in a rather standard way. A psychiatric social worker would see the parents to take a social and developmental history; a child psychiatrist would see the child once or twice; and a child psychologist would test the child with a mixture of intelligence, attainment and projective tests. If the child was then recommended for psychotherapy, a child psychotherapist would meet the parents for one consultation before beginning the child's treatment which could vary from one to five times weekly sessions. The social worker would offer regular sessions to the parents. This model gradually disappeared, as a consequence of changes within professional structures and identities – psychologists became very doubtful about the usefulness of testing; social workers wanted to become therapists and not to be the handmaidens of other professionals; and child psychotherapists came to be seen as competent to assess for treatment except where there were evident medical factors. The traditional professional family, one might say, where the psychiatrist as father exercised overall authority, was replaced by a more democratic conception of teamwork, which allowed the different available professionals to contribute their varied expertise.

What emerged were multi-disciplinary assessment teams, where the likelihood was that at least two of the available professions would

 DOI: 10.4324/9781003325543-10

be represented in work on any case. The senior clinician might come from any of the disciplines, though the choice would take into account what we knew from the referral information. For example, if there was a strong element of school difficulties, an educational psychologist might take on the case consultant role. If the child was in care to the local authority a social worker would probably be the first choice. This pattern is based on our experience that liaison with external agencies is often best managed by those with a deep familiarity with their practice and a shared language. This proved particularly important in doctor to doctor communications. I am going to provide some clinical examples demonstrating this model of work. When I work with cases on a single-handed basis I try to sustain the multi-layered thinking which a team approach facilitates, while being aware of the pull towards a focus on the individual, since that is my own clinical specialism.

A major shift in practice occurred when first interviews began to involve the whole family or at least the parents and the referred child. Involving fathers from the outset was intended to avoid the trap of designating emotional problems within the family as "mother's business", and the likelihood that an absent parent would represent a split-off aspect of family functioning of which we need to become aware. I usually prefer to meet first with parents alone if the child is a young one, and with the child first if he or she is adolescent. The fundamental aim of the assessment interviews is not to diagnose but to explore with the patients how they themselves see their problems, to find out what help they are seeking, and think about which members of the family could fruitfully be involved in treatment. The aim is to offer an experience of being listened to, of working towards understanding and most importantly of joint responsibility for this process.

I am going to describe briefly three ongoing assessments which will highlight some of the inherent variety of this work. They cover a spectrum from a case where psychoanalysis for a child is both needed and sought, a case where there remain a number of issues to be clarified, to a case where attention to the child's external circumstances is the pressing priority and the possibility of psychotherapy needs to be considered within a wider context of recommendations.

The first case demonstrates the appropriateness of a referral for psychotherapy, but also the reluctance that parents may have to pursue this path. The story begins two years ago, with a request for help from a professional couple in relation to their younger daughter Jessica then aged seven. They wrote of their concern about her reluctance to acknowledge her femininity, her troubled sleep and the tensions in her relationship with her mother. I met first with the parents. Father is aged 70, a distinguished-looking, upright but elderly figure, still working in his academic field. Mother is a teacher in her mid-50s. Her face conveys a gentle and sensitive nature, but also shows lines of deep worry. There is an older girl, aged 16. Father is British and mother was born in Africa, but Jessica spent the first three and a half years of her life in Canada, only returning to England after that. Mother's own mother is unwell, and there has been much journeying to and from Africa in recent years.

When I met Jessica, she turned out to be a slightly boyish and immediately eloquent child, very eager to talk about what worried her. Her anxieties centred on overwhelming aggressive feelings which she felt she had to conceal from her parents, but more seriously on her difficulties in distinguishing between fantasy and reality. She spoke at length about a film, 'Home Alone', which had engendered severe panic states. She was aware of being unable to see the difference between the characters in the film and some of the adults of her everyday world, and was terrified by the idea that benign appearances could disguise murderous realities. In our two initial sessions Jessica gained considerable relief from my understanding of her, and her anxious behaviour at home lessened. I recommended to the parents that psychotherapy be arranged, but probably in part due to the cessation of severe symptoms they decided not to pursue this immediately. Mother wrote some months later to tell me that Jessica was much calmer, but I was not altogether surprised to hear from them again subsequently.

The new problems concerned a crisis at school. In January, the teacher of her class had disappeared unexpectedly, to be replaced by two others. There was an atmosphere of mystery about the old teacher, who I was informed had in fact been dismissed following complaints of unsatisfactory performance, which had originated with a child in the class. Jessica does not dislike the new teachers, nor does she have a realistic difficulty with the work, but she has become extremely anxious about going to school, and when there she has great difficulty in staying in the classroom. She wakes very early in the morning, tense with fright, complains of headaches and tummy pains, and fights about getting in and out of the car. In school she runs out of the room, and even out of school altogether. The teachers have been sympathetic, and have devised a supportive structure for her. When she cannot bear the class she is allowed to go and sit by the headmistress's study, and she also meets the headmistress once a week to talk about how she is managing in school.

I arranged to see Jessica. She was brought by her mother. This time the extent of her boyishness was a shock to me. She had a boy's haircut and I at first thought I was looking at a boy in the waiting room, where she was playing with another younger child. She came with me as I explained that I now had a new room, which is in fact larger and more comfortable, but her first comment was about the slight drip from the tap in the sink in the corner. When I asked her to tell me about the difficulties at school which her mother had written about, it was very hard to hear much of what she said. She seemed deeply depressed, talking in truncated phrases, avoiding my eyes, sitting slumped in her chair. With a good deal of gentle encouragement she managed to convey how frightened she was, and that she does not know what it is all about. She tries hard and knows it cannot go on like this. She has got to go to school, but she feels sick and wants to scream. When I get home, she said, by this time talking more confidently, I get very fierce with my mother. This struck me as an odd word in this context, an adjective more commonly used of wild animals than of cross or angry children. I found myself feeling very worried about her mental state, and also sensing the helplessness and panic about which her mother had written.

She described how difficult it was to go to sleep. She wakes very early, feeling ill, is tired all the time and doesn't get any lunch at school because she can't join the other children. She told me she did not understand why the teacher had left, and puzzled over the half-explanations she had been offered, demonstrating both an effort to be rational and her sense of defeat.

She then lapsed into gloomy silence as if she had told me all she could, and I was struck by my own paralysis of mind, wondering how we would get through a 50-minute session. With relief I found myself noticing one sign of life. Her hands were at play. Each was holding on to an arm of the chair, with the fingers playing out a rhythm. I could not catch what it was but wondered aloud if it might be a musical message. She became more animated and responded with a comment and a change in her posture. She pointed out a dent in the arm of her chair. She wondered how it had got there.

There was a similar but smaller indentation on the other arm. She felt these delicately with her fingers, exploring them in detail. They were not in quite parallel positions she noted. The second development was her moving her two hands towards each other across her body until they met, fingers slowly extended towards each other and finally touching, but only just, conveying a feeling of the two hands not quite matching as the arms of the chair did not. Jessica measured the chair-arm slowly, and told me one was longer than the other. As I talked to her about these thoughts about the chair, about my room with its leaky tap and not-quite-right chair, the atmosphere lightened and her voice strengthened and regained its ordinary pitch. She showed me that on one of her hands two fingers feel stuck together and so the hand as a whole cannot work properly. We had a conversation about her belief that something inside her has gone wrong. She developed the finger game, scratching the ends of the chair-arms with her nails and telling me that she was smoothing them to make them feel the same. The ambiguity of whether she was scratching off varnish and damaging the chair, or relieving her anxieties about difference, misfit and the impact of the passage of time by trying to smooth away the evidence seemed clear.

At the end of the session her despair and desperation expressed themselves dramatically. Her voice again faded to a whisper, and she told me her father cannot help. "It can't go on like this", she pleaded. "I'm frightened about going to school tomorrow. It's getting worse, what can I do?" I said I would see her again next week, and we would think about what would help her.

It was evident to me that the urgency of being able to convey her sense of not being able to cope was carrying not only the present burden of misery and anxiety but also the knowledge that my previous proposal of therapy had led nowhere. She was telling me this time something must happen. "You must take this seriously" was the message to me. My understanding was that this girl's deep vulnerability to depression was a consequence of three factors. One was the extent of her aggressive impulses. The second was the inhibition of reality-testing, due to her anxieties about her parents' capacities to tolerate hatred and other negative emotions. The third is the probability that she may face the loss of a parent or a partial loss through illness at a much earlier age than the average child. Her father will be well over 80 by the time she reaches adulthood. She seemed to me to lack the internal resources to deal with significant loss, and analysis could help her with this. I thought it likely that her tomboy-ishness was related to these issues. A mother who may be deprived of a potent husband will have, instead, a lively boy; a female self too identified with a damaged internal mother is defended against by the overdevelopment of a boy self who denies involvement. This split in her echoes the over-intense, burdened worry of her mother, and the somewhat unreal denial of ageing, vulnerability and passion in her father's slightly bland and over-rational personality. I think that Jessica has unconsciously chosen a symptom her parents will not take lightly. Both value her education greatly, and are very upset by all these difficulties at school. It should therefore prove possible to arrange therapy for her at this point. She can thus be helped with those aspects of her personality that her parents cannot contain.

This kind of case might be seen as a classical example of the appropriateness of child analysis. Here we have a child in great mental pain, who is seeking understanding of herself, has an awareness of internal reality and its power and potential for meaning, and parents who are likely to understand the reasons for treatment. One would hope too that some opportunity for Jessica's parents to be seen alongside Jessica's therapy would enable them to understand more and be better prepared for the complexities of the adolescent years ahead.

My next clinical example is perhaps more representative of the majority of cases referred to child and adolescent services. The question of how to frame the intervention is more obviously problematic with a need to keep more than one track in focus. A letter from Ms T requested help with her younger adopted child aged 22 months. I wrote to offer an initial consultation and she phoned immediately to accept and to ask whether she was expected to bring her son to the session. When I returned the call I left a message that I would prefer to see her alone on this first occasion.

Ms T is a single parent with two children adopted from a Central American country, Teresa aged five and a half and Pablo, now three. She is a pleasant-looking, informally dressed woman in her early 40s and has a professional practice in complementary medicine.

She began to cry in her second sentence as she told me about Pablo who she fears must have been sexually abused as a baby because his behaviour towards her is so strange. He backs away from her when he wakes up to the corner of his cot, hiding his face behind his hands and arms, and screaming. She does not know whether to pick him up, or leave him. But stranger than this is his attitude towards her body. He pokes his finger repeatedly into her umbilicus, her mouth and the hollow in her neck beneath her chin. Then he retches or vomits repeatedly. She feels he is seeing vaginas everywhere, and gradually investigating all the orifices of her body. In her home, she is relaxed about nudity, which would be very different from his home country where bodies are never uncovered. She now wonders if her naked body reminds him of some abusive experience, though he does not show any other sexualised behaviour.

I said that it might be best to think about these things with her once I understood a little more about the children's history. She was then able to tell me her history. Finding herself unable to conceive or to sustain a relationship, and having always wanted to have children, she decided to adopt. As she believed she would have difficulties in being accepted as an adoptive parent in London she decided to consider a country where she had lived and worked during the 1980s. Because of her powerful cultural link and her commitment to bringing up the children bilingually, she was accepted. She adopted Teresa, aged ten months, and immediately bonded with her. Teresa was tiny and malnourished, but began to make up lost ground quickly. Then Teresa's mother told Ms T about a half-brother, and she eventually decided to offer him a home too, feeling it would be so good for Teresa. Pablo had been terribly neglected, strapped into a chair all day, his head misshapen as a consequence, with little stimulation and very little food. He had been cared for by his grandmother, in great poverty.

In contrast to the experience of immediate attachment to Teresa, Pablo did not call forth her maternal feelings, and she was finding it very difficult to adapt to the new shape of the family. There had been much anxiety about his physical health. At first he suffered severe muscular spasms, which were frightening to behold, though these were thankfully diagnosed to be a consequence of protein deficiency and have now ended. He has also had two episodes of grand mal (his natural mother is epileptic), which have been investigated and may indicate epilepsy, though the EEG is at present normal.

Ms T spoke clearly, though with evident anxiety about how much harder it was to be a single parent than she had ever imagined. She knew that having Pablo had been the most wonderful thing she had ever done for Teresa, but she was very concerned that she herself would not love him in the same way.

What issues emerge from this initial consultation? A number of areas of concern are indicated. The most worrying was the risk of rejection of Pablo. I learned almost as an afterthought that the adoption was not yet legally completed. Ms T was clearly under great strain in trying to reshape a family to encompass the three of them. When I asked about her own family of origin, I heard that she was the middle of three sisters, but she said nothing of her parents. Because of Pablo's many physical problems he had already been referred to two specialist children's hospitals, with well-known child psychiatry departments. In each of these, mother had been reassured by the predictions made about his development, and had felt unable to convey the relationship difficulties, which were for her so much more pressing. The same pattern had been repeated during her visits to the Well-Baby Clinic at the Anna Freud Centre, where she had not found it possible to draw attention to the seriousness of her worries. She had felt not helped but frustrated by the remarkable recovery and growth of her handsome little boy on which everyone complimented her. While being told repeatedly how well she was doing, what frightened her was awareness of her lack of feeling for the child.

The unconscious hatred of this little boy who threatened to disrupt the symbiotic link to Teresa became more evident in our second session. This over-close relationship to Teresa suggested that psychic separation had not been achieved between them. She felt that she and the child were physically joined in a state of perfect mutual understanding and delight. It was however interesting to hear when I saw mother for the second time that she was feeling a bit fed up with Teresa's clinginess. She explained that Teresa follows her around like a shadow and sometimes this strikes her as oppressive. We could then begin to discuss whether she could envisage space for adult friendships or for a lover in her life.

Another area of concern for me was the position of Pablo in relation to his masculine development. One could hypothesise that his urgent communication of sexual curiosity and excitement was not only warning his mother of his need for more physical boundaries and protection from over-stimulation, but was also a demand that his otherness, his little boy nature, be acknowledged. I think it is likely that Ms T may be uncertain about her sexuality. She has perhaps retreated from heterosexual disappointment to a life within a community of single women and children. In such groups aggression is perceived to lie with the excluded adult males. For little boys growing up in this atmosphere it can be very difficult for their potency to be experienced positively.

I am aware that I have emphasised the family dimensions of the problems Ms T presents. However, I also viewed these exploratory consultations as an opportunity to help her towards psychotherapy for herself, which I thought she might be ready to seek. She seemed to me to be a brave person, willing to take on the psychic implications of her life decisions. I was impressed by the fact that in our second meeting she was no longer so focussed on problems seen to reside in Pablo's present behaviour or past and forever unknowable history, and was more balanced in her perception of her two children.

What can and should be done for the children? One option would be to refer the mother for psychotherapy and trust to that to modify her projections and thus to create a proper space for the children's growth. However, I think there is a good argument for something additional, particularly in the context of her single-parent status. It is more difficult for lone parents to gain a perspective on their children; the triangular space created by a parental couple related to their child always contains multiple points of contact with dynamic potential. I thought the consultation with me had provided a glimpse of this extra dimension, allowing Ms T to withdraw some of the hostile projections into Pablo, and to take some distance from Teresa because she felt supported by our ongoing conversation. A second reason for undertaking further exploration of the children's situation is the extremely complex circumstances in which these children are growing up – two cultures, two languages, two mothers, an absence of paternal figures. My experience of work with adopted children and their families suggests that even a straightforward adoption brings major psychological tasks in its train. An inter-country adoption where the vision of the abandoned and deprived mother is perpetually revisited is inevitably a complex undertaking.

I therefore proposed to Ms T that I meet next with all three of them, so that I could get my own sense of the children's personalities. My expectation was that subsequent to this I could hold a watching brief, maintaining a link with her as a parent, of which she can make use if need arises. One might surmise that either or both of the children might need help at some point. In the meantime Ms T can be referred for therapy in her own right. She had in fact herself realised that the reason she wanted a second appointment was that she feared my eyes would turn towards the children and that she would feel neglected. This capacity for contact with her own infantile self was a positive indication for psychotherapy.

My final example is one where family life has broken down; Lee, aged 11, is a child with an absent family. He lives in a children's home together with his older sister. The referral to the clinic requested advice about the suitability of placing brother and sister together in a foster home, and about possible psychotherapeutic treatment. Such an assessment is complex in its scope and aims. We decided to work as follows: an initial meeting between two child psychotherapists and the children's social workers, two joint sessions with both children and both therapists, two individual sessions for each child; a feedback meeting with the social workers to discuss possible action. Large resources are required for this sort of work, but our experience has demonstrated repeatedly that unless both the legally responsible social worker, and those with day-to-day care of the children are involved in the clinical process, splitting between the professionals takes place and either the assessment itself or the following through of recommendations is subject to sabotage. Children who have experienced multiple disruptions and betrayals by adults project their picture of the adult world into the professionals who try to cooperate for their benefit, and the processes of projective identification make it extremely difficult for us not to re-enact the children's despairing expectations.

I shall now present one of the individual sessions with Lee. In the joint sessions his sister had seemed a good deal less damaged than he. She seemed ready for foster placement. He presented a more worrying picture. Here is a summary of the session.

He arrived ten minutes late with his social worker. In the waiting room he was arguing with her, and ignored the arrival of his therapist, then detached himself completely from her, and offered his hand to the (male) therapist. As their hands touched, he drew his hand back sharply, as if he had received an electric shock, but he then reached out again. In the room he took out a 50 pence coin, and laid it on the table. Later he mentioned that this was to buy a drink. He then took a ball from the toybox and proposed a game of catch. This was the game his sister had initiated in the previous two sessions.

He then began to build a zoo, but abandoned it half-completed. He took out a man doll, a car and an ambulance. The man fell, as if hurt. The ambulance was coming for him but it took a long time and when it arrived the man was run over. The man doll was then put in a truck instead.

The play sequences changed frequently with no apparent rationale, and in the next few minutes all the dolls ended up being shot, and Lee talked about a war yesterday. The therapist became aware of something peculiar about Lee's eyes. The two of them appeared to be looking at each other, but their eyes never quite met.

Lee then picked his nose, turned his back and ate a large mass of mucus, despite the therapist's offer of a tissue. The new mucus was spread on his face and clothes and he seemed to become more and more inaccessible.

Then he began to play again with the animals and a fight took place between a mother kangaroo and a tiger over a baby, who got mauled and eaten in the course of the fight. The therapist talked to Lee about his experience of people fighting over him, perhaps Mum and social workers. The therapist was doubtful if Lee was listening to him.

At the end of the session Lee insisted that he could find his own way back to the waiting room, but immediately turned in the wrong direction and then twice tried to enter the wrong room. He disengaged from the therapist completely, and did not say goodbye.

The distressing picture of Lee we gain from this is probably painfully familiar to those of you who have worked with children who have suffered multiple rejection and loss and are at the mercy of a world which fails to protect them from emotional abuse. Lee's problem in developing any trust in adults is continuously amplified by their failure to support him. Even in these crucial assessment sessions the residential social workers repeatedly brought the children late and they were brought by different people each week. Lee's mother, who has several other children in care and a new baby at home with her, cannot provide any consistent input for the children. She often fails to turn up for her agreed weekly visits. Lee and his sister are nonetheless attached to their mother. Previous attempts at fostering have broken down partly because of her involvement, and partly because of Lee's very difficult behaviour. He is unpredictably aggressive towards other children, manipulative with adults, and he smears faeces around the house. He is also unable to attend school.

In the session we can see the unconscious beliefs underlying Lee's behaviour. He attaches himself promiscuously to whoever is at hand, but at an adhesive, surface level, without an expectation of relationship. His mistrust is vividly demonstrated as he first offers and then withdraws his hand. His only sources of comfort are material: money is a resource he knows how to get; his own body products are there when there is nothing else. The despair is evident in the depiction of the ambulance as the source of injury, not help, but so is the active turning away from what might be offered. Lee has a squint, but took off his glasses at the beginning of the session and left them lying on the floor. The previous week he had left them in the taxi which brought them to the clinic. He has moved towards perverse activities from which it is difficult to detach him. There is some evidence of the capacity for symbolic play in the fight over the baby, but he shows no visible interest in the therapist's effort to explore meaning. His omnipotent claim to need no help, to already know his way about the clinic, provides a taste of how difficult this boy must be to educate.

We found ourselves considering the following options. It seemed clear that Lee would quickly break the hearts of any ordinary foster family. The motivation of foster parents can only be sustained by some positive capacity for attachment in the child. A therapeutic community placement seems a more realistic option, where the painfulness of the child's rejection of help can be shared between workers with a support system to help them to bear it. Individual psychotherapy could be (ideally should be) one aspect of such a placement. The link to his sister, his only lifelong attachment figure, is, however, important, and any plans for placement need to include arrangements for them to have regular and reliable time together. It is always extremely difficult to get agreement to a plan of this sort, because of the great cost of therapeutic community placement.

A second option might be to find a specialist foster family with experience of such unrewarding children and with parental resilience. This could be combined with arrangements for Lee's education in a "Special School" (a few of these remain) and outpatient psychotherapy. As far as therapy is concerned, I would tend to offer once a week for some months as an extended assessment of Lee's capacity to make use of it. If a tolerance of meaning shows signs of developing, the frequency of sessions could then be increased. I do not think we should underestimate the futility and damage that unrealistic efforts at therapy can engender. Inexperienced therapists can be deeply undermined by such patients, the children themselves, if unready for it, may lose the chance of approaching it more usefully at a later point.

One should take note of the difficulties that would certainly emerge in any attempt to provide psychotherapy for a child like Lee. Such has been the undependability of the adult figures in his life hitherto that a therapist's own reliability and commitment would soon be put to the test. Lee's aggression and degrading attitude to his own body and to shared space would be likely to create very difficult problems of management for his therapist. My experience suggests that this would challenge the institution in which the therapy takes place as well as the therapist. He would try to make his therapist hate and fear him, as this would be the only way in which he might gain relief from his own horrible despair. This means that the treatment of such a child will reach to the depths of the therapist's analytic capacity. Even an experienced therapist needs time to recover from sessions with a child like this, and opportunities to talk to colleagues. A less experienced one would need good supervision, in particular to address the enormous problems of processing the countertransference. The consequences of unreliability in the support of the therapy – for example in missed sessions or lateness – would be likely to be experienced as cruelties by the child, and thus visited on the therapist too. Work would therefore be needed with the carers to enable them to understand the absolute importance of maintaining the setting.

It is extremely difficult for us as therapists to bear the guilt of seeing children in such a terrible state for whom we may nonetheless be able to do very little, and in this we need the support of our colleagues. I think this sort of case can only be dealt with adequately if the therapists involved have an opportunity to discuss their work within a colleague group which can share the pain of this sort of responsibility.

SECTION 3

THE PARTICULAR NEEDS OF YOUNG PEOPLE GROWING UP IN FOSTER OR ADOPTIVE HOMES

8

MULTIPLE FAMILIES IN MIND (1999)

The structure of the internal world of adopted children and their families is influenced in many subtle ways by their atypical life experiences. This is also the case for foster children and parents when long-term placements are made. In this paper I describe how the complex internal worlds of participants in adoption dramas influence ongoing relationships within substitute families. This is an evolving process, and has a span beyond one lifetime because of intergenerational transmission. There is now a well-established understanding that adoption cannot be meaningfully understood as a one-off event or moment and needs to be seen as a process, whose meaning is reworked throughout the life cycle (Rosenberg, 1992). Individual psychotherapeutic work can offer detailed descriptive accounts of adoptive experience from the perspective of internal reality, thus taking account of unconscious elements, and this is the primary evidential base from which this paper is written.

A brief discussion of the concept of the internal world introduces the theoretical framework underlying the clinical approach described. This concept was Klein's (1946) major theoretical contribution. It elaborates Freud's picture of a domain of internal or psychic reality (Meltzer, 1981). Klein's work with small children introduced her to the concrete way in which children experience what she called 'internal objects.' These are the internal representations of the significant persons of the child's external world whose qualities will have been influenced by what the child has made of his or her experience.

The concrete quality of the small child's inner world, and of Klein's concept of unconscious phantasy is well exemplified in the following vignette (Isaacs, 1948). A two-and-a-half-year-old girl

DOI: 10.4324/9781003325543-12

who had been more or less toilet-trained became extremely anxious about defecating in the toilet following the birth of a younger sibling. She insisted on wearing a nappy while sitting on the toilet, into which she could then defecate. Eventually she was able to explain that this was necessary because she was frightened that the baby inside her would fall into the toilet when she did a poo. If she used a nappy she could check and be sure that it was poo not a baby that was flushed away. The 'realness' of the internal world was making it very difficult for this little girl to differentiate between imagination and external reality.

A second important feature of a young child's picture of the world is that it is only gradually integrated and organized. For example, the inner picture of a mother holding her baby, the representation of a cradling function, is gradually transformed into a picture of a more complex mother – arms that hold become linked to eyes that look at the baby, to a face that smiles, to breasts that feed, to a voice that speaks and sings, to the smell of mother's skin and so on. In a framework of good enough external care, the infant mind structures the varied fragments of experience and two pictures of mother take shape, one of a good trustworthy mother with all those attributes that gratify the infant, and a contrasting picture of a bad, unreliable and disappointing mother. This process is what psychoanalysis calls splitting, and it is a fundamental achievement in psychological development which permits us to organize our mental lives in a differentiated way. Good and bad, beautiful and ugly, right and wrong, love and hate, are primary polarities on which we depend to order experience (Klein, 1946).

As the baby develops, it becomes possible for a well-supported infant to perceive the connection between the good and bad mothers of the inner world. The baby can also begin to struggle with the task which occupies us all internally throughout our lives, that is the bringing together of our diverse and contradictory feelings towards the objects of our passionate feelings, and of partial pictures of ourselves. The growing capacity to sort out self and other is the bedrock of persons becoming individuals. It is interfered with when the care of the young child is not consistent enough to assist processes of discrimination and not attuned enough to the infant's needs to modify early infantile anxieties.

The care received in the early months or years of many of the children who are subsequently adopted is likely to have lacked these

126

helpful features. We need to bear this in mind when we try to grasp their experience of themselves and the impact they have on their new families. The care they require may be of a quite different order from that which their chronological age would lead one to expect. Their internal worlds are very often confused, lacking in meaningful differentiations (Boston & Szur, 1983).

Some features of multiple family life have a striking impact on the nature of the child's inner world. The markers of familiar places, so important to young children, may be confused or lacking. Sounds, smells, the view out of the window may have changed unpredictably as did the humans in view. There has to be space in the mind for not only birth parents and adoptive parents, but in all likelihood also for significant other foster carers who have provided periods of care. In addition, there may be an area of disorganized experience where individual carers did not feature strongly enough to acquire a recognizable shape in the child's mind. This can be a consequence of multiple indiscriminate care in an institution, of multi-adult disorganized care in a severely dysfunctional family or of the experience of being cared for by a mentally ill parent who did not seem to the infant to be a recurring recognizable figure. These examples are not exhaustive, but may serve to help us imagine a child's response to particular sorts of care. The social worker is an additional significant figure, and sometimes has provided the greatest continuity over a considerable period. The flow charts (Boston, Lush, & Grainger, 1991) which document placement sequence have been found most useful in working with adopted children. They have to be seen as adjuncts to the family trees which might be viewed as providing equivalent information in more ordinary cases.

Anxieties caused by 'contact'

Current practice often places an expectation on adoptive families of coping with a range of forms of contact with the original family. But this mental over-crowding can be disturbing to a child.

Katy, aged nine, in a recent conversation with her adoptive mother explained that she did not want any contact with her birth mother. Specifically, she did not want her adoptive mother to write the agreed annual letter to her birth mother giving a brief account of her and her brother's progress. She was very relieved to reassure herself that photographs were not being sent and she certainly did not want to send a card or note herself. Why not? Because, she anxiously confided to her adoptive mother, she feared that her birth mother might be able to trace her via her finger prints. Katy has recurrent nightmares that she will be kidnapped by her mother even though she has been in her adoptive home for a number of years and there is no contact.

It is as if Katy's sense of safety in her new family is intruded on quite out-of-the-blue by this figure of a mother–kidnapper. From Katy's point of view, the nightmare could always start to happen in real life. Explanation and reassurance about her position does not help her, for in her internal world she remains at the mercy of an all-knowing, all-powerful and terrifying mother. This is the legacy of the neglect and abuse she suffered as a small child feeling help-less in the face of cruelty. Sometimes her behaviour in the adop-tive family seems to have the meaning of an attempt to pass on this horrific experience of being explosively intruded into, as in her recent symptom of sudden long piercing shrieks, right into some-one else's ear. Katy is so frightened of these attackers that she is not able to acknowledge the reality of her own difficult behaviour – from her point of view, she is engaged in necessary self-protection. Sometimes she provides a glimpse of the simplified idealized world she seems to be in need of. Her current delight is in learning to canoe – the snug fit for one within the firm structure of the canoe, the special clothes and life–jacket, could represent the absent longed-for link to a caring sustaining mother, who holds the baby up above her terrors instead of plunging her into them. Katy's opportunity to achieve basic splitting into good and bad was probably undermined in her early development. This building block of the mind has to be in place before integration can occur. From greater integration can flow the capacity to take responsibility and to feel concern for others.

Small nuclear families are not particularly characteristic of humankind over the centuries. There is some sense in likening the linked network of foster homes created in some localities to the more extended families of other periods and indeed of some minority ethnic cultures within modern-day Britain. In some local authorities, the fostering support services enable foster parents to get to know each other and to provide respite care between foster homes to facilitate holidays and cope with crises in much the way grandparents and uncles and aunts sometimes support a family in need of help with childcare. What is difficult for these children is to get a grasp on what a mother, father, brother or sister is, when they have such a patchwork of broken-up experiences to draw on.

This element of confusion can further complicate the degree of conflict, particularly conflicts of loyalty, which such children often face. The crucial process of making sense of things, although it will in part be a conscious process, and can be assisted from outside by work of a life-story type and in other ways, is, to a significant extent, an unconscious process, taking place in the depths of the mind.

Contributions from clinical research

In exploring this matter of conflict, a research project by Deborah Hindle has yielded significant and striking data (Hindle, 2000). She used careful observational assessment of siblings in care, together with meetings with the network of adults involved, to examine the decision-making process with respect to siblings being placed together or separately, and to try to refine some useful criteria for such decisions. She worked with two sisters, aged three and a half and one and a half, who at that point were living in separate foster homes. This arrangement was a consequence of a judicial decision that rehabilitation of the older child with the natural mother should be attempted once more. When the child was again abandoned, she was returned to a different foster home, though contact visits with her younger sister were maintained.

When the children were seen together their play was animated. The older girl, Kelly, made many moves to include, refer to and take care of her little sister, Susie. When Kelly left the room briefly to go to the toilet, Susie flopped on the floor and remained huddled and lifeless until she returned. The girls used each other's names frequently. When Kelly was seen alone she was markedly more disturbed, and was suspicious of and hostile towards the therapist. The story stem technique developed by Hodges and Steele (1995) for research with children with disrupted life experience was used as an additional research instrument. Kelly's stories contained no evidence that she expected children who got lost or hurt to receive any help from adults, and threatening intruders seemed to be all-powerful, totally overwhelming the inhabitants of the doll's house. There was no model of a relationship imbued with concern between adult and child. Yet Kelly had been observed to provide quite tender care-taking for her baby sister – between sisters, something protective did seem to operate. When Susie was seen alone, there was repeated reference by name to her absent sister.

The conflict that this material highlighted was as follows: both foster mothers maintained that the child in their care had no memory of having lived with the other, and that the children did not know they were sisters. Kelly was said to have no particular relationship to Susie, 'She's like that with everyone,' said Mrs A, and Susie was said by Mrs B to have forgotten the time Kelly lived with them. Yet both foster mothers were identified with their foster children and protective towards them. How can we account for this sort of blind spot?

Each foster mother was perhaps fearful that a shared placement could endanger the interests of 'their' child. Mrs A was angry with Mrs B that Kelly had not returned to the Bs following the abortive attempted rehabilitation with mother. She perhaps carried Kelly's feelings of rejection by Mrs B and the failure to protect her from yet a further chapter of hurt. Mrs A had been enthusiastic at first to keep Kelly as a long-term foster child, in the light of her mother's refusal to free her for adoption (Susie had been given up for adoption at birth), but this optimism had waned sharply and she was now seeing herself as providing a short-term placement. She, too, was thus feeling unable to hold on to Kelly in the long-term and perhaps her guilt about this was pushed in Mrs B's direction.

Mrs B who had cared for Susie since birth knew that Susie was in pretty good shape, and that although as elderly foster parents she and Mr B could not offer an adoptive home, there was every chance that she would be placed in a good home while they might perhaps remain in a quasi-grandparental role. Thus, without the additional complications attached to Kelly's presence, in particular her not-yet-resolved link to her birth mother and to two older half-brothers, Susie could be seen as part of a new 'ideal' family. Kelly's presence would bring back into play all the uncomfortable elements in Susie's background.

There is an obvious disjunction between the evidence that the children's link with each other is of importance to them and the denial of this by the foster parents. One way of thinking about this is to note that the foster mothers' interpretation of the facts tends to reduce both the pain and uncertainty that the story presents. If we are in touch with the children's sense of investment in each other, it is very painful to imagine what each has felt about their sudden separation and it seems clear that maintaining their relationship is a priority. If we argue for a joint adoptive placement, we have to recognize that this will probably involve a delay in Susie's permanent placement and an element of risk, since Kelly might again evoke in a family an initial wish to have her, followed by an equally strong feeling of rejection. It is obvious that she is a little girl who will place great strain on any family's emotional resources, and that therapeutic help should be sought for her in conjunction with placement plans being made. All this means that the prospective adoptive family is going to need to be exceptional, and in particular, be able to accommodate two children who will easily offer themselves as stereotypical opposites – the nice and the nasty one, the responsive and the non-attached. The family would also need to be able to tolerate sharing the care of one of their newly adopted daughters with a therapist. This is rarely a palatable idea for adopters, who usually hope that the 'forever' family will do all that is needed to put right a child's problems.

Clinical intervention

Once humans get close to each other, their internal worlds are in a dynamic relation to each other. All the earlier experiences of each member of any significant intimate relationship (dyad, triad, family, group, etc.) contribute to the landscape of the new relationship. Events in the present can throw into prominence troubling aspects of the past, both providing a chance for a new way forward but also often engendering confusion and distress.

Clinical interventions take us to the heart of these complex interactions. My first clinical example concerns work with an adopted boy aged nine. In this case, the internal world of the adoptive mother became a powerful organizer of the child's developing personality. This intergenerational intertwining of unconscious imaginative lives can create particular quandaries within adopting families. In the second example the emphasis is on the process going in the opposite direction, the impact of child on parent. Both examples raise some of the cultural complexities so commonly associated with adoption.

First clinical example

Sam, aged nine, is the adopted son of a couple who have lived in England for some years. He was referred for help with severe sleeping difficulties based on an acute phobia of snakes. At the time he was unable to sleep alone and woke in panicky states several times a night. The parents were exhausted and at their wits' end. Other difficulties noted were his jealous relationship with his younger sister (also adopted) and his intensely combative spirit when confronted with parental authority. He seemed unable to accept that adults had any rights commensurate with their responsibilities.

I offered to see Sam once a week for psychotherapy after two assessment sessions in which he gained some immediate relief, but also gave me a sense of the entrenched defensive impasse which was being enacted at home. The GP had written of a brief focal intervention in relation to the sleeping problems, but I thought that something more extended was needed.

In the first term, Sam was reasonably communicative about all sorts of matters except anything that might pertain to the difficulties at home, of which I heard nothing. The parents continued to express extreme exasperation. Sam seemed very enthusiastic about coming to see me, using his time to the full, but for the purpose of interesting or occupying me rather than receiving anything from me. He would listen politely to what I said, but then brush it aside and enquire if he could now continue with whatever game he was engaged in. I struggled with growing frustration.

When working within a psychoanalytic framework, the therapist anticipates that the breaks within the regular treatment rhythm are of significance, because attention is being paid to infantile aspects of the therapeutic relationship and this usually means that separations have a major emotional impact. However, the extent to which Sam's way of relating to me shifted prior to the first holiday break was a considerable surprise to me as I shall describe. More often, we find that breaks acquire significance once they have been experienced. For children with earlier disruptions in their history, however, they may be felt as a repetition of earlier abandonments and make their impact felt before they have actually happened. This always seems extraordinary at the time, but in my experience the child is relieved when it is possible to speak about feelings suddenly erupting into the therapy from an unfamiliar area of the personality or from undigested aspects of personal history.

The last session of the term brought a dramatic shift. Sam was in the waiting room together with the rest of his family, tearful, turning away from me to hide in his coat and completely unwilling to come to my room. I decided to invite his parents to join us to get things underway. They both spoke volubly, while he remained slumped in a sad heap, and mother left after a few minutes to return to the younger sister. Father then spoke warmly about how proud he was of his son, who was now able to go to bed on his own and was not waking them up at night. This had the quality of both affectionate support of Sam, but also an implicit statement that he did not need to come to the clinic any more, and that therefore what was happening in the room was unimportant, and should be brought to a close as soon as possible.

After a while, I decided to ask father to return to the waiting room, saying that although we could both see how upset Sam was, I thought he could manage to spend some time with me on his own, and stating to Sam that if he felt this was not so he could return to his Dad at any time. Father left, a bit reluctantly, and I then felt free to speak to Sam directly about his feeling that I had become quite a different Mrs Rustin for him now that I was going to be away over Christmas and not seeing him for two weeks. He could not find the Mrs Rustin he had liked talking to here today. I said that I thought he believed that I was leaving him altogether, as his long-ago first mummy had done, and that he did not trust what I had said about starting sessions again in January. Sam was able to stay for the rest of the session while I talked on these lines, linking his mistrust with his worry that I would not remember him, did not like him, wanted to get away from him and so on. He quietened and relaxed, although still looking very miserable.

When we resumed in January, a long sequence of sessions ensued spent on building armaments of defences – planes, missiles, laser systems, ever bigger bombs. Numerous wars were enacted in which the enemy, linked usually with the enemies of his country of birth, attacked and was held at bay by the superior defence system so carefully constructed. Each renewed attack required an escalation of the security system. He told me that he wanted to join the army when he was old enough. His world picture was of his country standing alone, taking on the whole world and surviving by monumental efforts.

I began to describe to him that the 'no,' which became his virtually automatic response to anything I said, was like a kind of force field, a wall of 'noes' to keep me out, like the plasticine palisade he built around his camps. Occasionally he would allow me through for a second; a couple of times this took the humorous form of his saying 'Yes – I mean no' in response to what I said. Yet it seemed impossible to interest him in exploring these contradictions. I experienced him as almost impenetrable and could not see any way to convey to him that I might be able to help his beleaguered self.

I had tried on numerous occasions to make some link to the pre-holiday session, to no avail, but one day I roused myself to try afresh to locate the terrified and despairing Sam I had glimpsed just that once. Perhaps I spoke in a more imaginative way than usual as I described how puzzling it was to understand where that boy had gone, for Sam had been telling me repeatedly that he had no more problems now, echoing his father's words. Suddenly he looked up at me and said, 'That boy left. That wasn't me. He's in Hollywood.' Thus began the story of the boy in Hollywood. Sam explained that the boy rings him every day to talk to him. Next week I heard more. The boy does not have any more problems at night because his nanny, Jacky, has helped him. She stays with him until he falls asleep, but the boy is still worried about being on his own. He thinks if he snuggles down inside his blankets so that he can't see the snakes, he might be all right, but he's not very sure. Soon I learnt that the boy was getting very frightened because Jacky was going to leave to return to Canada – her sister was going to have a baby, and Jacky was going to help her. The boy was very sad indeed. 'I'll see her once more,' said Sam, quickly correcting himself, 'I mean he'll see her once more.' The boy supposed he would have a new nanny but he liked Jacky.

Now I will describe in more detail part of the session that followed this. Sam began by fetching his huge war-plane construction, made of ruler, pencils, Sellotape and plasticine, together with his remaining plasticine, which is what he used to make missiles. I remarked that today he had an idea of needing to check up on being well protected. I had in mind the closeness of the Easter holiday but did not refer to it at this point. He then produced a large bag full of 'pogs' from his pocket (there was a wide-spread fashion for collecting these little toy objects at the time), the metal type which are similar to large old fashioned half-crowns, embossed on each side.

Using the plasticine, he made what he called 'fake pogs' by imprinting them on the plasticine and cutting out matching rounds. He became more adept and drew my attention to how well the pattern came out. I talked to him about his wondering how well I would be remembering him over Easter and how well he might be able to keep me in mind in the weeks we did not see each other. I linked this back to the upset before Christmas, when he felt afraid I would not keep him clearly in my mind and would lose him and not come back to go on with our work. 'That was the boy from Hollywood,' he corrected me, but in a tolerant tone of voice which allowed our conversation to proceed. He then told me more about this boy when I enquired how he was. He was very sad and afraid since his nanny left; his cousin had been looking after him, but she would be leaving next week to go back to her family. I said I wondered if Sam could help that boy. He looked at me, a bit surprised. I explained that he might be able to talk to him as he knew something about being very upset when someone left. When I went away at Christmas he had been upset, but he also knew that I had come back, and that this was what would happen again at Easter time – we would say goodbye, but we would meet again after the holiday to continue our work. There was a brief pause and then he looked up and said he would see Jacky again one day. When he is 18, he will go to Canada to visit her.

Sam then began a game to see which were better, the real or the false pogs. He decided the fake ones were better because they were heavier and softer, more flexible. He showed me how they stick well to the pog they are thrown at and to the surface of the table, instead of just bouncing off.

I spoke about this making me think about his liking things that stick well, that don't get detached. I linked this with his feeling more hopeful about us sticking together, not bouncing off in opposite directions and losing contact. Then I went on to talk about his ideas about a contrast between his first mummy who had not been able to hold on to him, and his adoptive mummy who might feel like a fake mummy in one sense, because he had not grown inside her, but seemed to him to be better for him because she stuck to him. He said quietly 'my belly Mummy.' I asked was that his way of referring to his first mummy? 'No,' he said, 'it's my Mum's way. She doesn't like me to call my original Mummy my Mum.' I said it would be good for us to use the words he liked for thinking about her – was that his name for her? He confirmed thoughtfully, 'Yes, my original Mum.' I talked about his having lost her a long time ago but perhaps still having a lot of thoughts about her. Losing people that were important had started right at the beginning of his life. 'I was only two weeks old,' Sam said. 'My memory doesn't stretch that far back.' I agreed and added that in his imagination his original mum probably was still important.

There was some further reference to the idea of a new nanny and Sam thought I said 'Nana' and corrected me. I asked if he had a nana too. He was puzzled and I explained some people called their grand-mothers 'nana' and I had wondered if he did. He looked up and calmly summarized for me precisely described details of his mother's traumatic early history as the child of two holocaust survivors, and added a painful episode from his father's family history.

Towards the end of the session he began to crush together the fake pogs. 'How many of them are still alive?' he asked me, as if in a game. He showed me that it was still possible to disentangle from the lump of plasticine a complete fake pog with the image clearly visible.

I talked to him about memories of people who had died being still alive in people's minds, both his and his mother's. Perhaps this was also linked to his thoughts about his original mother – he might wonder sometimes if she was still alive. 'And her parents,' he added. 'People at school say I look like my Mum and Dad and my sister,' he said. I asked what he thought about that. 'I don't think I do,' he said. I spoke of his realizing that other people sometimes found it difficult to allow him to be a boy who had had an original mother and father and therefore tried to pretend that his family now was the only one he belonged to. He did not feel like that, and he wanted me to help him to think about the pictures he also has in his mind of his original mother and father.

He asked me if I still have the building blocks he used to play with. I fetched them for him. For the last part of the session he built constructions with rather substantial foundations which were in fas-cinating contrast to the tall, wobbly towers of the earlier period of brick play, which had always collapsed spectacularly. This building turned out to be quite solid at the base, and a good portion survived when he built a spindly top section obviously destined to fall over.

I talked about his feeling differently about coming to the end of the session today. I suggested he felt we had had a good solid talk and that even though finishing was difficult (as usual he was very slow about clearing up, in an attempt to prolong the session) he felt there was something which would remain there in his mind and in mine for us to build on next time – it was not all just a heap of fragments. Like a comic echo of this, as he picked up his jacket, he scattered coins all over the floor and grinned at me as he gathered them together.

Discussion

I shall explore three different threads in this material. Firstly, the story of the boy in Hollywood. I think it was crucial that I did not prematurely cut off this story-line. At a suitably great distance and for a brief time (London to Hollywood, the length of a phone call) Sam could make contact with the terrified boy within him. We could discuss the boy's fear that nanny and others left him because they were fed up with him and couldn't bear all his worries. We could picture the boy's wish to remember and be remembered and his great fear of being abandoned. Over a number of weeks, Hollywood got palpably nearer, and I think Sam needed to be allowed to manage the pace of this integration (Alvarez, 1992). It will probably continue to move back and forth. We have, however, found a place where terrible anxieties can be located and yet contacted.

The notion of the boy in Hollywood offers a way of working over anxieties which Sam needs to be able to externalize and hold at a distance. This manoeuvre is a creative solution to the problem of being easily overwhelmed by intense feelings. It would be unhelpful to interpret the projection and take away the space in which there is freedom for us to explore together.

This links to my second point. The horror of the mother's tragic history is spoken about by Sam coolly and rationally. Only a tiny hint of the emotional meaning of the holocaust is offered. When he told me later on in the session about his aunt, he referred to her ashes being in the wood where a memorial playground had been built. My mind registered the link between the crematoria of the death camps and his reference to his aunt's ashes in the forest. The interweaving of these images of catastrophe with the idea of children's play space provides us with a vivid sense of how little unimpeded space for play there may be in the family landscape of children whose parents are close to the holocaust. I think Sam's account conveyed to me how

137

laden down he is with his mother's tragedies, how much detail he has been burdened with, how much she may have needed her children's mental space for her own painful memories.

The family history he has had to ingest is not one he is able to imbue with real significance. The headline quality of his announcement that he was going to tell me his mother's tragic story indicates the distance between what is hers and what is his. This is of course one of the subtle difficulties in intergenerational construction of narratives of family history, for the teller of the story has a particular inflection and point of view, and an adult view tends to crowd out the child's perspective.

The third point is that we are shown Sam's pained distance from other people's version of his life. He must have got across to me in his tone of voice that the phrase 'belly Mummy' was not quite right for him, as I think I questioned him in response to this half-perceived note of discomfort. More explicit was his complaint about the pressure he feels in the school and social world to go along with the fiction of a perfectly fitting family of four. This fiction involves disloyalty to his emotional link to his birth mother, and in so far as that link is weakened he is also more exposed to the impact of his adoptive mother's traumatic history. I found myself thinking about the possibility that some of Sam's angry rejecting behaviour towards his mother may be a desperate effort to hold her at a distance and protect himself to a degree from being sucked into her nightmares. It is interesting to see how much he has been helped by a nanny who is more able to respond to his need for an understanding of his fearfulness because she herself is not so easily stirred into states of panic.

We have here a dramatic representation of the traumata of the earlier generation which have not been digested in the mind or found symbolic representation. Probably the nightmare black snakes are in some way linked to Sam's picture of the horrors of death camps which his mother needs him to help her to deal with – perhaps associated with black leather Nazi gear or the black columns of smoke from the crematoria or with swastikas.

Let us consider the parents for a moment. Mother's capacity to contain and process her own appalling experiences have been further damaged by her inability to bear children. This may have made her feel that the Nazi curse had got right into her body, destroying her fertility. This additional loss, after so many early ones, sets the scene for the adoption to carry an enormous weight of hope and anxiety – if this parental couple can come together, the hope is that the nightmare of the holocaust can be set to one side and an area of new growth be established. But the dread of a repetition of disaster is extreme, making both parents ill-equipped for the ordinary ups and downs of raising children. Every reverse is experienced as the beginning of a destructive process which cannot be controlled. Hence Sam's tempers are described as quite overwhelming for both parents who each try to leave the other one to cope alone.

Second clinical example

Now what about the parental perspective? I have chosen an example which offers a glimpse of the processes of working through anxieties which have a double resonance, an echo for both parent and child. I think it shows how the fresh opportunities for dealing with fundamentals raised by our relationships with our children can lead to moments of resolution and change.

I am working with the single mother, Ms B, of an adopted 17-year-old boy who has had a very turbulent delinquent adolescence. Steve currently lives in an excellent hostel, and this physical separation has contributed to considerable rebuilding of their relationship. One day mother described to me the events surrounding Steve's birthday. They had gone on a shopping trip together to buy him new clothes. She had set a cash limit which had been made explicit to Steve, and which, as always, was generous in the context of her limited resources. To her delight, Steve had chosen items within a manageable price range so that he had a complete new outfit with which he was pleased. They had a snack together. As they were to say goodbye at the bus stop in Oxford Street, Steve tried to extract from her the few remaining pounds up to her cash limit for the birthday gift. She refused, feeling flooded with anxieties about what he wanted the money for (usually drugs or debts to dealers), and with rage at the way in which her generous present was now being made to seem mean. Steve's threats and verbal and physical abuse of her escalated, to the numb astonishment of the many bystanders, and to the despair and horror of Ms B who felt herself reliving a hundred previous violent rows. Steve screamed among much else 'No mother would treat a son the way you treat me. You only think about yourself – you're not my mother, you bitch.' She managed to escape with the arrival of her bus, arriving home still shaking with fury and terror and having retaliated with this reject-ing parting-shot – 'I don't want to see you for two weeks, Steve.'

Later, she calmed down, and thought to herself, 'I can't do that. It's his birthday. He's had enough of being abandoned by people. I'm his mother and I can't not be there on his birthday.' She then left a message for him at his hostel – would he like to arrange something for his birthday? If so, please will he let her know. (She was think-ing maybe go to a movie.) Steve responded – can they have a meal together?

In this sequence of passionate emotions stirred so strongly by the particularly painful edge associated with birthdays for adopted chil-dren, things get out of hand, but each of the two struggles hard to avoid a repetition of the so-well-rehearsed breakdown of relation-ship, and thus to allow that the present can be more than the past repeated. Something new is always a possibility. Without this ele-ment of optimism, adoption could never have been invented as a solution to something that has not worked. But the complexity of the task never fails to fill me with wonder.

Conclusion

It is a lifelong reality for adopted children and their parents that their lives will be affected in unpredictable ways by the earlier experi-ences of the child. This may be particularly difficult to comprehend when there is patchy knowledge of the child's early history – bad times may erupt in ways which are deeply puzzling, since there is an absence of ordinary family memories which help to make sense of things. This is one of the reasons why a proper provision for post-adoptive support for families is so important. The shadow of earlier turbulence is liable to fall on the family when developmental pressures are felt and when anxieties beset family members. Separa-tion, divorce, illness and death are a special threat to children whose inner security has major fault-lines, but ordinary changes – going to secondary school, moving house, new siblings arriving and leaving home – can also arouse intense worry. Adolescent sexual develop-ment, with its accompanying questions for the adopted child about the nature of the sexual couple which gave him life, is a particularly threatening time. Such preoccupations are often expressed through sexual relationships dominated by unconscious re-enactment of phan-tasies about birth parents, and this can be a particularly troubling time for families. Their experience of the complexities of negotiating their children's adolescence can thus be interwoven with a stark encounter with the meaning given by the adolescent to his early history, which may feel alien in distressing ways.

The essence of the matter is that adoption and fostering create extremely complex familial structures; the internal reality of this is the dimension I have mainly attempted to describe here. Changing legal and social frameworks frequently ensure that the external dimension, the ongoing real experience of contact with the original family, is increasingly part of the picture. Understanding the interaction of these two dimensions of phantasy and experience is a continuing challenge for the families and all who work with them.

9

CONCEPTUAL ANALYSIS OF CRITICAL MOMENTS IN THE LIFE OF VICTORIA CLIMBIÉ

A response to the Laming report (2003)

In this paper, I draw on a number of concepts I have found useful in reading the important and deeply disturbing report into the death of Victoria Climbié produced by Lord Laming (The Stationery Office, 2003). Victoria was a West African child sent to Europe in the care of her aunt, Kouao. She died as a consequence of cruelty and neglect at the hands of her aunt and her aunt's boyfriend, Manning, in particularly extreme circumstances. The failings of the statutory services which Laming's report revealed have been the basis for substantial legal and administrative changes in child protection policy.

Some of the concepts I make use of in my analysis are very close to everyday ideas. Others are drawn from psychoanalytic theory because I believe it illuminates the puzzling and repetitive facts revealed by the Inquiry. I shall pay particular attention to issues of mental pain, borderline functioning, infantile persecutory anxieties, confusion, defensive splitting and mirroring processes. The inadequate responses of individuals and institutions are, I argue, profoundly linked to the disturbing impact of what they are trying to manage. My thinking derives fundamentally from my practice as a child psychotherapist. Trying to understand and describe Victoria's state of mind during her time in England is at the heart of what was missed, and central to grasping the meaning of what happened. While aware of some of the social work literature, my main points

142   DOI: 10.4324/9781003325543-13

of reference derive from a clinical perspective, and are therefore in a somewhat more personal register.

Avoiding mental pain in child protection work

It seems essential to begin by paying attention to the central importance of the *mental* pain which all the individuals referred to by Lord Laming faced in their lives and work. Much of my commentary concerns the way in which ordinary professionals doing difficult work may deploy defences against mental pain. It is notable that while repeated emphasis is given in the Inquiry Report to the appalling nature of Victoria's physical injuries, there is little description of the mental agony she must have endured. No photographs can document that, of course, but I suspect that understanding the way in which mental pain is faced or avoided is crucial to making sense of the defensive evasion by large numbers of professionals which the report details.

What is it that, at root, is being avoided? I think a significant component is the psychological impact of becoming aware of Victoria's dreadful life circumstances. Defences against such awareness are much to the fore in the story reported, and defences against recognising reality necessarily involve severe distortions in the mind's capacity to function. Of particular relevance are frequent examples of 'turning a blind eye' (Steiner, 1985), that is, failing to see what is before one's eyes because to do so would cause too much psychic disturbance, and various forms of 'attacks on linking' (Bion, 1959), the systematic disconnection between things which logically belong together, again a defence which is employed because to make the link would be a source of painful anxiety.

In psychoanalytic theory, these two forms of defence are frequently found to predominate in individuals with what is known as borderline pathology, and this fact alerts us to the massive level of disfunction which Lord Laming's report depicts in social services, the health service and the police with respect to child protection work. Laming is clearly delineating organisations which might be described as functioning in a way analogous to the borderline patient (Rustin *et al.*, 2003), organisations many of whose staff, at all levels of seniority, are unable to face reality and operate as a consequence in ways designed to protect them from the catastrophic impact that they unconsciously believe a proper confrontation with reality would engender.

Psychoanalysts have described this form of defensive organisation in individuals in various ways, but one of the most useful conceptualisations has been by John Steiner. He named the protective structures created by the individual who is dominated by fear of reality as 'psychic retreats' (Steiner, 1993). Just as the individual patient can persuade himself unconsciously that reality can truly be avoided if he stays put within the narrow confines of his personal psychic retreat, so workers within the organisations described, and the organisations themselves as represented by their structures and practices, seem to have been convinced that they could escape having to think about their contact with Victoria and her aunt, Kouao. Thinking involves the attribution of meaning to our experience. Without a sense of meaning, it is difficult to imagine what personal responsibility for actions would amount to, and it is just this phenomenon which the report continually highlights.

The nature of the mental pain associated with borderline defences is specific: it concerns conflict between opposing forces, ultimately the forces of love and hate, and the guilt aroused by awareness of ambivalence. I think it is helpful to bear in mind that many of the actions (or moments of inaction) described in the report as obvious evidence of incompetence relate to the desire of professionals to keep a distance from the intense feelings stirred up by exposure to human cruelty and madness. The fear and hatred people felt is very occasionally hinted at.

Another disturbing and shocking theme is the level of dishonesty among witnesses. The everyday gloss on this is likely to attribute to the liar a conscious desire to escape blame. That is part of the story. It seems clear that evidence had been removed from various files with an explicit intention to deceive, and Lord Laming implies that some senior managers who changed their jobs after the tragedy may have been up to something equivalent. But the concept which may help us to understand more about what happened at the front line is that of unconscious mirroring between clients and professionals. Kouao's statements to the people who tried to help were full of both confusion and lies. It is often not at all simple to tell the difference between malicious dishonesty and the kind of confusion about truth which is part of borderline psychotic states. Kouao's behaviour during her later trial strongly suggests that her mental state was severely disturbed during this period; a serious personality disorder would be the probable diagnosis. The evidence of the report is that the impact of *her* confusion and distortion of the truth seems to have invaded the minds of many of those who came in contact with her, particularly once there was a relationship in which she was trying to get the other person to see things as she saw them. It is remarkable to observe just how successful she was in this aim: doctors, social workers, police, clergymen and others were frequently acting on the belief that Victoria had something wrong with her. This was variously identified as a disease (scabies), behaviour problems (enuresis and other disturbed behaviour) and possession by an evil spirit, but in all instances the problem was agreed to be that Victoria needed to be cured, and the bad thing inside her got rid of. Such was Kouao's conviction, and the power of her vision continuously obscured the facts. I believe that processes of projective identification, in which the thinking of the professionals was taken over by elements of Kouao's madness, go some way to explain how this can have happened. Instead of being able to observe and thus question Kouao's belief system, workers began to mirror it (Britton, 1981), as I shall describe.

Finally, the report causes one to ponder on the infantile anxieties which the tasks of child protection evoke in staff. Feelings of helplessness, of dependence and deference to authorities, of not knowing enough, of sticking to rules mindlessly like a terrorised child (indeed like Victoria herself in her observed behaviour in Kouao's presence), of fear and of wanting to return to the 'normal' world as soon as possible predominate. The kind of training and support made available to staff does not seem to have helped them to mobilise more adult mental capacities to cope with the unavoidable emotional disturbance of this difficult work.

The report

Before moving to a more detailed exploration making use of the concepts I have outlined, it is helpful to be reminded of the report's contents. The 400 pages of the full report have an impact on the reader which is more than just the labour of reading such a dense text. The report deals with the background, including the story of Victoria's life in so far as it is known, and the contact with five different social work agencies, two hospitals and two police child protection teams. It also includes a brief section with reflections on issues of race and culture, carefully entitled 'Working with Diversity'. It describes a number of seminars in phase two of the Inquiry held to explore child protection work and their conclusions, and it makes a large number of recommendations to central government about social care, health care, policing and the broader governmental framework supporting the care and protection of children. There are 108 recommendations. They are predominantly directed towards improvement of procedures and of the supervision and management of all the services involved so that there can be confidence in the idea that the procedures will be followed. This arises from Lord Laming's repeated observation that poor practice was the root of the problem – established procedures were not followed, social work, police and hospital procedures, procedures for interagency co-work, for record keeping, for supervision of junior staff. My interest lies in elucidating why such widespread failure might be taking place, and I believe that it goes beyond the inefficiencies, system failures and personal mistakes the report describes. The recommendations are mostly very helpful in setting up a system that would remedy the management and organisational deficiencies if we were simply dealing with matters of good organisation and sensible practice.

But from time to time the report notes such things as 'if she had applied her mind to the matter' (13.41) (referring to Victoria's unexplained injuries) or 'The concept of "respectful uncertainty" should lie at the heart of the relationships between the social worker and the family'. Such comments refer to a difficult domain, to the individual worker's thinking about the case, and to the unavoidable anxiety of allowing such thinking to take place, in particular, anxiety linked to uncertainty and exploration. This is the area of professional work most easily interfered with by anxiety, both professional anxiety related to the culture of organisations (e.g. about inadequate resources for doing the necessary work, about fear of blame) and anxieties arising from close contact with the difficulties of clients.

Victoria's story – a deeper look

There is a great deal that can be added to Victoria's story as presented if we allow our minds to gather the significance of some of the details. The photograph of Victoria at the beginning of the report shows a child who was seen as a source of pride: her clothes and hair are immaculate, just as Kouao is always noted to have been very well turned out, in marked contrast to the shabby and neglected presentation of Victoria as the months went by. This picture of a child who could inspire interest and affection comes across in reading the account of her stay in hospital only seven months before her death. It is evident that within this child was a lively capacity for an affectionate and appropriately dependent relationship with adults. She attached herself to a French-speaking nurse who had been asked to spend some time with her with the enthusiasm and trustfulness of a small child whom life has not scarred. Perhaps her pleasure in visiting the neonatal ward was connected to her memories of her younger siblings and a community with many children around. But we can observe that this goes alongside her recent and ongoing experience of life with Kouao which clearly gave her a very different picture of the world.

How could this child keep these two grossly divergent forms of relationship so sealed off from each other? The familiar account in the child abuse literature is that the child's shame and guilt about what is going on, together with the fear of the abuser, enforces secrecy (Summit, 1983). We might add to this the suggestion that Victoria may well have shared in a phenomenon frequently seen in 'looked after' children, namely the great difficulty in bringing together the different worlds she felt part of (Rustin, 2001). The world of her childhood home with her parents in the Ivory Coast and her life with Kouao diverged so utterly. Then there is the time in France and her move to England. In France, Kouao's other children were present – they then disappear, along with school, a known place and a familiar language. On top of this are the frequent moves of house – bed and breakfast short-term arrangements, child-minding in yet another unfamiliar home, and later the arrival of Kouao's boyfriend, Manning, on the scene. Given Kouao's evident disturbance, we also have to try to imagine the hour-by-hour uncertainty of Victoria's existence.

How does a child manage the absence of any solid point of reference in place or persons? We get some clues about Victoria's response to this. She was, I think, terrified of abandonment. Her anxious state when left, after admission to the Central Middlesex Hospital, by the daughter of Mrs Cameron, her child-minder, is a clear example of this. This fundamental fear played a part in her frantic efforts to please Kouao by her behaviour. After all, Kouao had taken her to Mrs Cameron's on one occasion asking that she stay there for good.

'Do I belong anywhere and will anyone look after me?' must have been Victoria's silent question. The decision of her parents to send her as the 'favoured' child to Europe for the supposed educational benefit is bound to have had a complex meaning for her. On the one hand, she is the specially good and intelligent girl who gets the special chance; on the other she might well feel at an unconscious level that she was the one who was not wanted at home. 'Why me?' must have been a worrying preoccupation. This background is important in grasping her acute anxiety about being attached to somebody, and also in understanding how she would be unable to reach out for help by telling someone what was going on. I think she feared that a 'bad' Victoria was the unwanted one. The hospitals which discharged her so inappropriately may have added to her fear that there was no one who could bear the bad Victoria. The appalling combined onslaught of Kouao and Manning, which relegated her to a position altogether outside humanity, must have continuously sapped her capacity to believe she was worth anything to anybody. Manning said 'she wouldn't cry' when giving evidence about the daily beating of Victoria. I think we might say there was no one she believed would hear her cry, in the sense of giving meaning to the pain she was enduring, but also no longer a part of herself that could feel or think anything other than that she was an unendurable sub-human creature. The destruction of the personality, which has been described so well as a very frequent concomitant of concentration camp torment, comes to mind (Levi, 1958).

Lord Laming writes that in the last few weeks of her life, as she lay in the bath in an unheated bathroom, in her own excrement, cramped, weak, starving and wrapped in bin liners, Victoria might have been 'desperately hoping someone would find her'. I think this is an optimistic interpretation. Victoria had not been able to make a claim for rescue when she was in a much less deteriorated state. It is important to allow ourselves to acknowledge that hope can be destroyed, because when something like this has happened we long for protest, but the victim may be beyond that, and trapped in a world of nightmare.

The problem of identity

A vital detail in the story, in my opinion, is the meaning to Victoria and Kouao of the fact that her name was changed in her passport to fit that of another child Kouao had intended to bring to Europe,

'Anna'. One's name is a core element in a sense of personal identity and having to pretend she was 'Anna' will have played a part in Victoria's loss of sense of self and worth, and her confusion and anxiety. Added to this is the extraordinary fact of her shaven head and wig, intended to make her look like the girl whose photograph was to be seen in the passport. We have to imagine what this might have felt like to Victoria: her very self is being denied in such traumatising acts. Also important is the evidence that Kouao really had had *another* child in mind. We know from recent research quite a lot about the way in which a child who is perceived as a replacement for a lost child may be at risk (Etchegoyen, 1997), and Victoria was undoubtedly a 'replacement' child.

However manipulative Kouao's wish to have a dependent child who would give her access to housing and welfare benefits, I think it is necessary to consider the idea that Victoria not actually *being* Anna was a problem with more than practical significance for Kouao. She made efforts to involve the church in her problems with Victoria: was the 'Victoria' element perhaps seen as the source of the diabolical possession which had to be driven out by prayer and exorcism?

Victoria's symptoms

In the Inquiry Report, Victoria's urinary incontinence features as the supposed source of Manning's wish to get rid of her. What might this behavioural symptom have meant? There is no evidence of previous incontinence, and there had been medical oversight during her stay in France. At that time, her problems were described as exhaustion and a skin infection. I think we can surmise that Victoria's capacity for holding on to her feelings was stretched beyond bearing by the accumulated stresses of the chaotic weeks alone with Kouao. This child, apparently, did not cry but she leaked urine, which may have represented her unshed tears. Incontinence in a previously continent child was also a warning that she was breaking down. Her capacity to hold herself together had given way.

We cannot know what Victoria felt when Kouao and she moved in with Manning, but some hypotheses suggest themselves. Kouao and Manning's sexual life and interest in each other, rather than her, was displayed to her as they all slept in one room. It is possible that this was the first time Victoria was with Kouao while she was involved with a partner. In France, the story is that they shared a

149

home only with Kouao's older children. The vision of a couple must have evoked memories of her parents which may have been very upsetting, particularly in the context of her increasingly horrible daily experience. A child with a memory somewhere of loving parents, but a current experience of parents like our worst nightmares, is under terrible strain. The grief and rage at her abandonment by good parents must have been immense.

Incontinence is not an easy symptom for ordinary good parents to deal with. It stirs primitive anxieties about contamination, bad smells, about something that can go on and on and overwhelm the capability for absorbing mess and cleaning up. The sodden mattress that was eventually thrown out is an apt metaphor for the collapse of containment in the increasingly deadly interchange between Victoria and her tormentors. Her expressions of hopelessness and helplessness through her incontinence probably provoked their sadism to ever greater extremity. Their crude efforts to protect themselves from the increasingly catastrophic mess and the contamination they feared was, I suggest, the basis for the ghastly imprisonment of Victoria in the bathroom and in the bin-bag. She had become, for them, dangerous rubbish by which they felt persecuted. The absence of appropriate concern about these symptoms, at least partial knowledge of which was shared between a number of people, suggests to me that others had been disturbed by what they knew in ways they were unable to process. Easier to push it out of sight and out of mind.

Listening to the child

Another recorded feature of Victoria's behaviour is the occasion on which she shouted at the social worker in terms which made it pretty clear that she was echoing her aunt's line of argument. Victoria said 'words to the effect that she (the social worker) did not respect her or her mother and that they should be given a house'. This is a child for whom English is not a first language who spoke on this occasion with urgency and clarity. The report discusses the idea of Victoria being coached to play her role, but we might also ponder some of the other resonances of this exchange. Victoria is herself the victim of extreme absence of human respect – she has been passed off as 'Anna' and is joining in the fiction that Kouao is her mother. If we hear her intervention solely as the way in which she is used as a mouthpiece for Kouao, we are missing the way in which she is also communicating about her own situation. She is a child in need of what most children see as the basic requirement for life – a house, a place to be.

This observation leads me to reflect on one of the facts of the contact with Victoria on which Lord Laming commented strongly, namely that she was never spoken to on her own, when privacy might have allowed her to convey more of the truth. In the formal language of the report, she was not 'interviewed' alone. Perhaps the very idea of 'interviewing' helps us to grasp why this was never done. It sounds so formal, and the word has forensic overtones. What a gap there is between the skills that social workers and others might have in interviewing adults and what might be needed to establish appropriate communication with a young child. The professional observations of Victoria which bring her most alive as a child are the few which record her time in the North Middlesex Hospital. In the earlier events, what Mrs Cameron the childminder had to say and what a junior doctor in the accident and emergency department noted are straightforward descriptions in everyday language of probable non-accidental injury. This was the diagnosis proposed by the first paediatrician to examine Victoria. He described her as 'very secretive', on the basis of an examination of Victoria conducted when Kouao was not present. This makes it clear that Victoria was not easily able to use the opportunity of people being concerned about her to reveal what was going on, even when her injuries were the immediate focus.

A capacity for communicating with children is expected of social workers and of police officers involved in child protection, but this is by no means an easy task for at least two reasons. The first, made worse by the absence of adequate training and supervision, is the inherent difficulty for adults who are virtual strangers to a child to find a way to talk, watch *and listen* which is appropriate. The deficit in skills in observing children's behaviour and interactions and in interpreting these is a serious issue (Tanner, 1999; Youell, 1999). However, even a large effort to improve this state of affairs, urgent as this is, will not deal with the second matter, which is the inevitable problem for a child to trust unfamiliar adults and for the adults to feel they can infringe the ordinary expectations of family privacy and interfere in the relations of children and their parents. Victoria's 'secretive' presentation makes it clear just how much

151

delicacy and persistence would have been needed to get through to her effectively. It is easy to be harshly critical of the professionals who failed in this task and compare them unfavourably with the untrained but more perceptive non-specialists. The non-professionals felt able to use their common sense, to notice things and accord them significance.

Without the involvement of teachers or others in the community who know a child over time, the professional task of child protection is up against exceptional odds. This fact also alerts us to identify the group of children who are most at risk, namely those about whom there is no such ongoing knowledge. Victoria's experience, like that of many refugee and asylum-seeking children, is that they had to join in deception in order to be safe. Victoria had to agree to be Anna at immigration control, for example. How could she do otherwise? Sorting out who can be trusted is a more or less impossible task for children in this sort of situation, and 'the authorities' are not in the least likely to appear trustworthy. The most basic authorities in Victoria's life, her parents, had after all unwittingly handed her over to her tormentor.

There is another feature of the story which merits comment. During their time in a West London district in which they were seeking housing, a social work duty officer recorded details of Victoria's appearance and described her as 'looking like one of the adverts you see for Action Aid'. In Victoria's mind she may indeed have come to see herself as someone who was a recipient of 'Action Aid', appalling as that had turned out to be. By this time she had deteriorated from the bright smiling child of the portrait to a state of neglect so extreme that she could be seen as the sort of child a charity would photograph in order to elicit sympathy and guilt in the Western world. There are two perspectives to keep in mind here – Victoria's own identification with being such a desperately needy child, and the problem for the professionals faced with the impact she had on them. There is not enough of anything available to offer to such children – not enough housing (hence the urgent wish to send them back to France) but more broadly not enough of human or material resources to allow ourselves to take in the extremities of deprivation that such children remind us of. The first social worker involved noted to herself the difference in skin colour between Kouao and Victoria, and the fact that Kouao did not comfort Victoria when she cried, and wondered whether they were indeed mother and daughter. Her inaction in the face of her doubts was, I think, related to the problem of how much awareness of deprivation she could allow into her mind.

Victoria's ethnicity and the political context

This touches on the major issue of what part in the tragedy was played by Victoria's ethnicity. Was her black skin a source of fear to some (linked to the theme of contamination discussed earlier) and also an excuse for politically correct but mindless thoughts about cultural differences in child care which could set to rest the alarming observations of her terrorised obedience when Kouao was present? Did it set in train, along the lines of the 'Action Aid' comment, unmanageable anxiety and guilt about just how many children might want help from London social service departments if they once got a chance? The whole business of the disputed diagnosis of scabies is another dimension. This diagnosis played a part in further inflaming the near-paranoid and uninformed responses within Haringey when the mention of scabies led to a refusal to visit by police and social services. That particular decision, when the duty of child protection got turned on its head into a conviction that staff needed to be protected from the child, is stark and shocking. To understand it, we must try to keep in mind the background of widespread hostility to immigration and the near-breakdown of more benign wishes to offer asylum in this country. From this point of view, the mixture of feelings evoked by the task is very difficult for individuals to manage. They are official representatives of a community which both desires to exclude and close borders, and yet tries to believe in its own generosity and good intentions. It is a hard business to make sense of such contradictions. The wider political atmosphere is a pressure which needs acknowledgement, not least because of the sharing of responsibility that this involves.

It was estimated, for example, that in the London Borough of Ealing 60–70% of referrals to the Intake team might be families coming from abroad. Alongside this striking statistic, which underlines the extent to which particular localities bear the brunt of such problems, the statement was made that 'there were not very clear protocols and guidance for dealing with people that were presenting from abroad and presenting as homeless . . . quite often I felt that people were left to rely on professional judgement'. Clearly the sense of vulnerability that workers feel when 'professional judgement' is what they have to turn to is acute. I think this expresses the loneliness and sense of exposure of individuals functioning without the protection of protocols. They are left to face the pain and deprivation in the context of severely limited resources. Lord Laming's procedures are not going to protect social workers or others at the front line in the community from the pressures of being aware of their limitations and of the extent of distress and deprivation in our society. Good training and supervision which could support thinking about painful experience would, however, modify the strain.

Feelings, communication and the avoidance of thought

The feelings aroused in doing this difficult work are hard to make space for. They are uncomfortable, and they are liable to cause trouble in the sense of demanding more thought and more work if they are taken seriously. They are the 'gut feelings' referred to by one witness who spoke about how these feelings got put to one side rather than be subject to reflection and evaluation. This fact is closely linked to the much-noted absence of any useful supervision of the work undertaken and in similar vein the absence of adequate detailed written notes at many crucial points. Not talking about and not writing down disturbing observations are examples of the avoidance of thought. In particular it was rare in this case that two minds got together to think about what was going on. The very many people involved seem to have had pitifully few moments of sharing their thoughts. This is obviously a system failure, but it is also a mirroring within the system of the multiple disconnections in Victoria's situation. There is a failure of linkage between the family in the Ivory Coast and her aunt, a discontinuity between the Ivory Coast, France and England, not to mention how many moves there may have been within any one country. There are also the two languages, which the peculiar beliefs surrounding the need for interpreters made worse. It was evident that Victoria understood and spoke a fair amount of English and that Kouao's capacity to function in English was dependent on what sort of hearing she felt she was getting. Yet the sense that communication could not be attempted because understanding might not be easy was recurrent.

Wherever one looks in the story, there is a sense that the message is not getting through. This applies to the conversations not held or not recorded, to literal messages not reaching their intended recipient and, at a more metaphorical level, to the fact that the meaning of what was going on was not grasped. Nobody 'got it', or at least nobody with the authority to act. The whole system ended up as powerless as Victoria, unable to make any sense of what had happened to her. For her to have access to her own life story, or in more formal language a capacity to convey a 'coherent narrative', would only have been possible if she could bring together in her mind utterly discrepant modes of experience.

At the level of rational discourse it is easy to say that joined-up thinking and collaborative practice are required for better child protection work. For Victoria, such integration of her mental life probably faced her with the dread that the badness would destroy the good completely. It may have felt safer to keep them completely apart in consequence. During her hospital stay, she could be at ease in the care of the nurses, but they saw a different child when Kouao arrived. Such extreme splitting is a defensive manoeuvre to protect the self from disintegration. Some similar processes were at work in the minds of many others whose everyday work and sense of reality would have been put at risk if the contradictions of the evidence and the professional conflicts had been faced up to. Lord Laming comments that the police had allowed themselves to be 'led by the nose' by social services. It is unsettling to realise that Victoria's parents and Victoria had been similarly 'led by the nose' by Kouao. There are numerous observations about Kouao's 'manipulative' behaviour which do not seem to have helped people to be especially alert to the dangers of reproducing such behaviour in the interprofessional network.

Mirroring

The concept of mirroring is a tricky one, and is certainly open to misuse and overuse. However, I think it is unavoidable that we note the extent to which the behaviour of professionals seems to have been distorted by their contact with Victoria and Kouao. In the report's introduction, mention is made of the tendency of 'those who deliberately exploit the vulnerability of children . . . go to great lengths to hide their activities' (1.14). When one goes on to read about the forgetting, the absence of notes and indeed the active destruction of evidence which emerged during the Inquiry, we can observe a plethora of people covering their tracks in various ways. One telling event was a long fax recording Victoria's admission at the Central Middlesex Hospital. It was handwritten and substantially illegible when finally received at the North Middlesex Hospital. No one followed up the indecipherable evidence. The extraordinary fact that people reported not being able to read the fax mirrors how at a much broader level people were not able to read (in the sense of interpret) the facts before their eyes. A further disturbing echo is that the mobility of staff and the numerous locum arrangements in front-line services render staff much less likely to be able to cope with the troubles of families who are themselves dislocated. In the case of children being looked after by local authorities, my clinical experience strongly suggests that continuity in the social work input is one of the best indicators for a better outcome. Homeless families, even more so if they are new arrivals from abroad, must be similarly in need of a constant focus, a point of reference, a face that becomes recognisable. It is very hard to provide this in large bureaucratic organisations, but the less we do so, the more we are likely to fail to work effectively.

Child protection and adult mental health

There has recently been considerable focus in the world of mental health policy-making for children and families on the high levels of risk faced by children growing up with a mentally ill parent (Department of Health, 2003). It has been widely observed that staff trained to deal with adult mental health problems often pay virtually no attention to the impact on the children of their clients of long-term exposure to disturbed and disturbing behaviour. Sometimes even the existence of dependent children in the household is ignored. This wider picture is relevant in thinking about Victoria's experience. As some of the less guarded descriptions of Kouao make clear, she was a frightening person to be with. Her comprehension and intelligibility varied greatly, her story was not coherent, and her demands aroused anxiety and guilt. The combination of her borderline functioning, her marginal social situation and her religious beliefs, including the idea of possession by an evil spirit, placed her squarely in a minority group with ideas very far from the

156

mainstream. This rendered her strange and hard to decipher. Added to this was the evidence of her partial knowledge of the law and her rights, always an unsettling and threatening situation for an anxious professional.

The episode in which Kouao involved Victoria in claiming to have been sexually abused by Manning captures the essence of the problem. Staff seem to have been so relieved that the accusation was swiftly withdrawn, and they were let off the hook of investigating suspected child sexual abuse, that they were not able to perceive the worrying implications of this sequence of events. Victoria's story of abuse did not have the right focus and never sounded right, but a child making a false accusation, whether put up to it by some-one else or not, alerts us to the fact that they are in trouble. Here again, the difficulty in hearing the underlying communication is evident. What needed tackling did not fit the procedures laid down for investigating child sexual abuse. Following up the case would have involved literally finding Kouao and Victoria, who had gone missing. The whole situation at this point was much more messy, chaotic and confusing, and did not fit under a tidy label.

The concept of child protection is so all-encompassing if we interpret it broadly that it is easy to see why all the pressure would go in the other direction. Protecting Victoria would have required an interpretation of the task which extended very broadly indeed. Each time workers managed to put aside the reasons for worry-ing about Kouao, they probably experienced something akin to the many moments in Victoria's day-to-day existence when she momentarily escaped being the focus of persecution. Getting out of the line of fire by compliance or by deadening herself to awareness and feeling, and staying out of touch with memory and hope, must have been cumulative.

Conclusion: training for mindfulness

Mindlessness is a defensive solution which unfortunately fits all too well with complex bureaucratic systems. In an individual person, the failure to keep things in mind, to make connections and to have a perspective that connects past and present is readily seen to lead to a fragmented sense of self and to disrupted relationships. Some of the individual workers who gave evidence sadly seem in their practice to have been functioning in this way. The absence of thoughtfulness is just as much in evidence at the level of systems. The combined impact of Victoria's and Kouao's states of mind, which I have tried to delineate, is very painful to absorb. Unless workers have a theory and practice which allows them to perceive such levels of distress and have a context in which they can assess its impact on them, instead of being pulled into identifications and counter-identifications, the casework required cannot be done. The nature of the training, ongoing supervision and consultation that are required is something that needs urgent attention at the many levels I have tried to explore in this chapter.

PSYCHOANALYTIC WORK WITH AN ADOPTED CHILD WITH A HISTORY OF EARLY ABUSE AND NEGLECT[1]

(2018)

Introduction

The institutional context for the case I shall discuss in this chapter is an important one and records an important moment in the development of child psychotherapy in the UK. The background in theoretical developments within Kleinian and post-Kleinian thinking is equally important, and I shall first address these two aspects of the framework which together made clinical work of this kind possible.

In the 1960s, courageous individual child psychotherapists began to attempt psychoanalytic work with children with very severely deprived and compromised early life experiences (Boston, 1972). This was a time when hopefulness about the potential impact of analytic work with severe disturbances in children was at its height in the London psychoanalytic community. There was considerable enthusiasm for child analysis from informed parents and child psychiatric colleagues, a growing demand for training, and a National Health Service network of clinics employing the still tiny number of qualified child psychotherapists to which a wide range of children in difficulties were being referred. The inherited wisdom of the child guidance tradition had been that "milieu" therapy (Dockar-Drysdale, 1990) was needed for children whose start in life had not provided a relationship with a "good enough" object. Psychoanalysis was

DOI: 10.4324/9781003325543-14

deemed to require an already established internalised good maternal figure as a starting point.

Bion's elaboration of Klein's account of the early development of mind (Bion, 1962b) was immediately seen by child analysts and psychotherapists to offer them something vital. His theory of maternal reverie, that is, the openness of the mother's mind in her care of her baby to receiving awareness of profound infantile anxieties and her capacity to transform these "nameless dreads" into meaningful emotional experience, described how a mind was formed through a relationship with a more mature being. Her attentive and attuned responsiveness formed the building blocks of meaning and thinking. The language of container/contained (Bion, 1970) made sense of the chaotic, unpredictable behaviour of young children whose anxieties had not been contained or given meaning in contexts of disorganised, neglectful, or abusive early parenting. Projective identification, thus reconceptualised as communication, and not only as intrusive and aggressive, opened up a new vista. If the fragmentation and intensity of these children's experiences could be "gathered" (Meltzer, 1967) in a transference relationship it seemed possible that development could be set in motion and their pathological defences be replaced by states of mind that would enable them to benefit from relationships, to grow, to feel more bearable emotions, and to learn.

This new psychoanalytic vertex required new techniques – classical interpretation of anxieties and defences was not tolerable or useful to patients whose minds could not yet conceive thoughts. The thinking and "dreaming" in Bion's terms about the earliest infantile fears as described by both Bion (1962b) and Bick (1968) had first to be done by the mother or, in the clinical context, by the analyst. This kind of realisation also led, for example, to Steiner's (1993) formulation of "analyst-centred" interpretations as the necessary precursor to interpretations that focus on the mind and experience of the patient.

Prior to many of these theoretical formulations, Bick's invention of infant observation (1964) for child psychotherapists at the start of clinical training had already proved to be immensely important in helping therapists find a way of being with children whose unformed minds were fragmented or liable to melt-down. The discipline of closely observing the emotional interchange of mothers and babies and of not intervening was a good basis for sustaining observation under pressure, and of receiving what a child needed to project without rushing to give it back. The patience and mental space needed to take in and hold on to what was being communicated, often in nonverbal ways, was a capacity that infant observation nourished and supported (Rustin, 2016). Child psychotherapists were therefore particularly attuned to the theorisation deriving from Bion's insights, eager to link their clinical and observational experience with his conceptualisations.

The Tavistock Clinic in the 1970s played a particular role in this evolution of clinical practice with children. The strong tradition of infant observation (Rustin, 2009), the clinic's commitment to work towards *national* mental health, meaning the population as a whole, not only the privileged minority who might have knowledge of and access to psychoanalysis, and the multi-disciplinary teams available to contribute to the care of patients led to the formation of a workshop. This provided an opportunity to study consultations to the institutions that were caring for severely deprived children – initially children's homes, and later mainly foster care – and to explore the potential for individual psychotherapy with these troubled children and adolescents (Boston & Szur, 1983). A large number of children were taken on for treatment and their therapy presented in the workshop, and this resulted in a growing conviction in the possibilities for internal change in the children. More understanding also took shape about the conditions that were required for this (long-term therapies, ongoing work with carers, close supervision to support therapists, institutional tolerance of much acting-out by the children, community liaison, especially with schools), and more understanding of the tremendous strain often placed on adoptive and foster families who gave these children shelter. There was also a keen appreciation of what a multi-disciplinary clinical research workshop could offer its members. The high levels of anxiety, mental pain, and uncertainty – and, indeed, in twenty-first-century terms, "risk" – that therapy with these children entailed, was contained by the structured process of the group's work. It supported clinicians taking risks in the best sense.

As child psychotherapy has gradually spread across the UK, one trend that stands out is the high level of referral of children in the care system for psychotherapy, and this remains one of the major ways in which public mental health clinics make use of child psychotherapists. Some modest but significant research work on process and outcome with this population has aided the recognition of the relevance of psychotherapy for children who have been neglected or maltreated in their early years (Kennedy & Midgley, 2007).

The case

The case I shall now discuss is probably fairly representative of many children adopted by parents eager to help those who have suffered a catastrophic start in life. Not infrequently, the families find that the children bring serious difficulties with them, which are very disturbing to their parents and others. My patient Tim was a boy aged eight when I began to see him on a once-weekly basis. This followed some months of intensive (three times a week) psychoanalytic psychotherapy with a colleague who unexpectedly became seriously ill. She hoped to return to work with him in due course, but this proved not to be possible. I therefore continued to see him, and the therapy ended when he was twelve and a half and had made a successful move into secondary school.

This case highlights some important contemporary issues in analytic work with children. The question of frequency is of course a very important one in psychoanalysis generally at this time. Although I only ever saw my patient once a week, I believe we had a psychoanalytic relationship. Despite the high level of acting out in his sessions in the early years, which I shall describe, it was possible to sustain a focus on transference/countertransference dynamics, and the work we did addressed deep levels of internal object relationships.

My patient seemed to lack a sense of belonging to the human family when I first met him. He had been adopted at the age of five, and his picture of himself as an outsider was painfully enacted in the family context. In his therapy, I felt pushed to extremes of anxiety and doubt about my capacity to hold on.

Tim's history

When Tim came to the P family at the age of three-and-three-quarters, he joined a family in which there was already one adopted son, Jack, aged seven at that time. The couple very much wished to have a family, and had decided they would adopt when it became clear that Mrs P would be unable to bear a child. In Jack they had already taken on a child with appalling early experiences. When a second boy became available for adoption, they agreed to go ahead, although family circumstances at that particular time were stressful and Mrs P was under a good deal of strain.

Tim's early years had been chaotic and full of tragedy. His birth mother was a prostitute, herself brought up in care as an adolescent. Her first child had been removed and subsequently adopted. Following several terminated pregnancies, she gave birth to Tim. Tim and she lived in at least six different places in his first three months of life. She separated from his father because of serious violence a few months later and the following year she married another man who was in and out of prison. He is said to have disliked Tim, who, however, seems to have had a special place in his mother's troubled heart. Another child was born in the following year, and Tim and his sibling spent numerous periods in local authority care on a voluntary basis. When Tim was two years old, there was a fire in their home and this little brother did not survive. Tim was taken into care and plans made for his future. She never gave her consent to his adoption, though she failed to turn up for the final court hearing, and so it went ahead.

When Tim came into care aged two-and-a-quarter, his behaviour in the foster family indicated a history of sexual abuse, which was investigated and broadly substantiated. At this time, he was described as being delayed in development: he had little speech, and could not feed himself. His behaviour was extremely sexualised, and he called everyone Mummy. His mother had weekly access visits. When she failed to turn up, Tim became obviously depressed. After more than a year in foster care, supported by a nursery placement, he had improved greatly and adoption began to be considered for him. However, when Tim went to live with the P family he became withdrawn; he avoided eye contact and regressed to indiscriminate behaviour.

Referral

When the Ps came to the Tavistock clinic some years later, originally because of their concern about Jack, they gradually began to share their worries about Tim. They described his secretiveness, his lying, his aggression towards other children, his sexualised behaviour, and later also spoke of their (particularly mother's) tremendous difficulty in getting close to him. They described their very first encounter with Tim when he was three and a half: he was roller skating along the pavement of a busy road at high speed, in the opposite direction from his foster home. Now aged seven, Tim would disappear if he hurt himself or felt ill and silently curl up in his bed. Mother felt wounded by this refusal of care, but later on was able to tell us that she felt she had not loved Tim when he first came to the family. In fact she said she had sometimes hated him: she felt so involved with Jack that there was nothing left for Tim. Father, however, felt closer to him. It is important to note here that consistent long-term support was provided for these parents by a very skilled psychiatric social worker throughout the period of their children's treatment.

Following the discovery of sexual play between the boys, Mr and Mrs P wanted therapy to be considered for Tim; Jack had already had one year's treatment. A psychotherapy assessment revealed Tim's extreme anxiety about his capacity and urge to destroy, but also gave a picture of a needy and expressive little boy. Some months later, therapy began on an intensive three times a week basis.

His first therapist had a very difficult two terms of work with him. After a brief seductive interlude, tremendous violence erupted. Tim wreaked havoc in the therapy room and disturbed his therapist deeply by his ruthlessness and inaccessibility. Unfortunately, she then became unexpectedly ill, and this entailed some months' absence from the clinic. What was to be done? Both Tim and his parents were in a highly upset state about Tim's therapy and its interruption, and it seemed necessary for the clinic to provide some holding for Tim. This is the point at which I became involved. I agreed to see Tim on a weekly basis until his therapy could resume.

Beginning therapy

In his first session with me, his challenging behaviour was immediately evident as he explored the room, attempting to poke holes in the ceiling tiles and to attract his brother's attention during his session, which was taking place at the same time elsewhere in the clinic, by semaphore-like antics at the window. However, he then became fascinated by the project of making a parachute. He used a small plastic bag that had contained some of the toys I provided for him, to which he fixed strands of Sellotape, linked together to represent an open parachute. He showed me that he wanted it to land gently, but anything he used to attach to the parachute turned out to be too heavy and to cause an immediate crash to the ground. He was both persistent and frustrated by the unsuitability of Sellotape for his purpose, and he left still intent on pursuing this idea and with a promise to try with string next week.

In the next couple of weeks he tested out my boundaries in every possible way, and also invented an elaborate game in which, he told me, I was to be trapped as a prisoner. The following session was missed due to a heavy snowfall that prevented the family reaching the clinic. When he next came, Tim began with a renewed interest in the parachute theme, which led me to talk about the shock of the missed session the week before. Perhaps, I suggested, it had felt like crashing to the ground when he realised they would not get here. His activities developed into a desperate effort to take control of the room and of me. This included a sequence in which he used the desk lamp to enact being an optician who then turned out to be a tor-turer, shining the light into my eyes and staring at me with a fiercely cruel expression. He was enraged when I turned my head away.

Turning his attention elsewhere, he crawled around under the furniture and the room was filled with a faecal smell. Next he tried to make a 999 (emergency) call on the telephone. Any comment from me elicited "Fuck off" or a snarl, with the exception of a brief interlude when he wanted to explain to me where he lived and drew a detailed map of the part of London where his home was. After I had thwarted his attempts to flood the room, he again became friendlier and started to tell me a version of the story of Cyrano de Bergerac in which his interest was focused on Cyrano's difficulty in getting a drink because his long nose always got in the way. I was able to talk to him about the idea that his intrusive nosiness about me and my room might in fact be preventing him getting something good from me.

In these early months of work there were many sessions that brought me to the edge of my capacities as a therapist. Tim threat-ened my peace of mind with a bewildering variety of weapons and I often felt close to hopelessness about being able to find the part of him that might respond to understanding. I would wake up on Thursday mornings, the day of his session, feeling very anxious and physically fearful – would I manage to keep things within some bearable degree of control? My fears ranged from his dangerous behaviour at the high window, with which he delighted in torment-ing me, to concern for my room and its contents and for my own physical integrity. These fears were sometimes realised, as when he held on to a handful of my hair as if to pull it out by the roots, but more often it was Tim's mental cruelty that left me feeling abused and exposed.

I spent large chunks of sessions feeling that I had nowhere to put myself – Tim would commandeer all the furniture and I would feel lost and homeless in my room. I experienced shame and helplessness, knowing that he would jeer at whatever I said, and felt huge and foolish. He once spoke of me as one of the smelly vagrants on the River Thames embankment, telling me I lived in a cardboard box; at that moment I certainly felt exposed to the cruellest elements of his personality in an unprotected way.

Later on in the work I came to better understand this experience of shame (Cregeen, 2009) when there was a session in which Tim enacted a sexual scene before me. He climbed on top of a high cupboard in my room on which he could lie full-length. Prior to this he had been scribbling abusive and sexually explicit words on the wall in red pen and he took the pen up with him, taunting me even more pointedly from above my head. As he lay there, I had to stand quite close to make sure he did not tumble down. As he writhed around in a state of wild excitement, he began to enact intercourse in a grossly lewd and noisy fashion, declaiming that I was desperate to touch him because he was so fantastic.

The horror and pain evoked in me was difficult to bear. I felt I was being made to feel what the toddler Tim had endured, an excruciating awareness of his mother's life as a prostitute to which he had been exposed, and simultaneously excited and humiliated. The mixture of his great love for her, and the ugly violation of her better self and his infantile vulnerability had, I believe, stirred up intense shame and confusion. The impact on his oedipal development of this premature exposure to adult sexual activity, doubtless heightened by the experience of actual sexual abuse, was alive in the room, and it was possible for me to speak to him about this. After describing what he was doing, I said that he wanted me to know about a little Tim who felt terribly upset when he imagined me in this room with a horrible Tavistock Daddy. He wanted to show me that his mind today was full of a sexy show-off Mummy – me, who enjoyed making him feel left out and forcing him to see things he could not bear. Perhaps there was a long-ago Tim who felt tormented by things Mummy did that he could not get out of his mind.

His response was very moving and unexpected. He quietened, asked me to help him climb down, and then fetched a cloth from the sink and washed all the red graffiti from the wall. He did this with extraordinary care and there was a deep silence in the room. It took him quite a long time.

Signs of development

I now want to describe some elements in the therapeutic process that represented his claim on a place in my mind. This gave him the feeling that he did belong somewhere (Rustin, 2006), even though this was a fragile conviction always easily disturbed by separations.

I think a degree of safety entered into Tim's relationship with me when he realised that the original idea of his returning to his first therapist was not practical and that I needed to continue with him on a long-term basis. Tim began to show me occasional searing glimpses of his painful memories. His vulnerability had always been evident whenever there was any possibility in our all-too-frequent physical struggles that he could be hurt. He behaved as if his skin had no solidity at all, and although at times I wondered if he wanted me to be guilty and anxious about the risk of hurting him, I mainly felt that he believed himself to lack any protective covering. In one session, after a long series of confrontations between us as to the limits of what I would allow, I held on to him as he stood on the desk by the window. Panting with the effort involved in preventing him from kicking me, I said to him,

Tim, one of my tasks is to take care of your body and of mine, not to let you or myself get hurt if I can prevent it. That is why I am holding you now, because you are not safe near the window when you are upset.

The fighting tension went out of his body and he curled up in a heap, crying very softly. After a few minutes he whispered to me, "Nobody ever took care of my body." I talked to him about his worries as a little boy that nobody cared for him, his belief that he could only rely on making himself feel big and strong to survive all the frightening things in the world, and his hope that I would understand all of this. I sat close to him, speaking very quietly, and with the conviction that my going on talking to him was very important.

He could not see me because he was curled up like a foetus, but I thought the sound of my voice was soothing to him, and that my words also would mean something.

At one point when I had been speaking of his baby experiences, he said very quietly "I don't want to talk about that any more now." On another occasion he had spent the first half of the session fighting me by hurling things from behind a barricade made of all the movable furniture in the room. Then he began to construct a camp inside this heap of furniture, using the blanket I provided as a roof. Curled up, completely hidden from me inside his safe haven, he communicated with weak cries and moans that he was starving and dreaming of food that was out of reach.

A crucial sequence of sessions took place after one Christmas break. Just before that holiday, he had been telling me with unusual freedom and pleasure about his school play, which was about convicts in nineteenth-century London who were to be transported to Australia. He was to play one of the convicts, and he described the prison ships and the farewell to friends and family on the last morning, and sang a poignant song about losing his homeland and all that he loved. He had a sweet singing voice and narrated this whole story with great feeling, making me think about the profound links between individuality and mother–infant communication (Malloch & Trevarthen, 2009). When he returned after the holiday, he had two sessions before his brother's therapy sessions resumed, and these visits to the clinic seemed to hold special meaning for him. His mother was bringing *just him*, not Tim merely as an attachment to the older child he believed to be the favourite. After a brief explosive entry, he looked around my room and suddenly it seemed he had a brainwave. He began to move all the furniture systematically into different positions, not in a jumble, but in order to create a quite new room. The physical labour involved in this was immense, and as I was concerned about the weight of some items, I offered to help him, which he accepted. We were co-operating like two furniture removers. He decorated the newly positioned desk with a plant and objects from his drawer of toys, which he said were to be ornaments, and created a little corner for himself, almost completely enclosed, where he could draw on the low table, kneeling on the blanket and pillow, while I sat and watched on a chair that he placed for me just by him. I had a conviction that Tim felt at home in a quite new way now that he had devised a way of making the room his own so dramatically. He began each of the following sessions by repeating this sequence.

One week into this sequence of sessions I received a message from Mr P cancelling all the family's sessions because of illness. Seven minutes after the usual start of Tim's session, I received a phone call from reception saying that Tim was in fact waiting for me: clearly there had been a muddle and the message given to me was wrong. I hastily prepared to receive Tim, which took a few minutes, and we therefore began about ten minutes late. Predictably enough, we had a terribly difficult session. He ran ahead and blocked me out of the room, and, in the end, I had to force my way in. There followed a long sequence of provocative and risky behaviours – spitting, hurling items, blood-curdling threats. The one quieter moment involved his playing with a wobbly tooth, eventually pulling it out triumphantly. Tim then immediately stared in a very anxious way at his tooth, convinced that he had pulled out some flesh with it and would now have what he called a "black hole" in his mouth. In the last few minutes of the session he turned my room into as big a mess as he could, maliciously commenting that it would take me a long time to clear up.

A crucial session

The following week started more calmly, and to my amazement we even entered the consulting room together, the first time this had been achieved in many months.

Straightaway but with a surly expression on his face, he began to move the furniture around. He accepted my help with the desk in quite a friendly way – negotiating which end to move, etc. – while I talked about his wanting to make the room feel his own today. The atmosphere seemed tense and volatile. When he moved towards the chest of drawers, he very violently slammed shut the drawer that contained his toys and materials. Then he bent to scratch at his leg just below the knee, a bit secretively, with his back to me. I wondered aloud if he might have a sore leg but be unsure about showing me. He came closer and told me, "It itches – it's a bite." I said, "When you want to bash and hurt something, the hurt seems to bounce back at you and leave you feeling hurt." Then he fetched the rug and lay down on the sofa, now under the window, and completely wrapped himself up inside it. Just as he was preparing to do this I suggested pulling the blind down as the room was getting rather hot. I decided to go ahead and do this, although it involved leaning over him to reach the window, which felt uncomfortably close. However, he remained peaceful. He briefly lay still inside the rug, then seemed to be scratching at something; I wondered aloud about what was feeling wrong. He replied, but I could hardly hear, and then he spoke again. It sounded like "shady and cool." I talked to him about his searching for protection from the sun, which felt too hot today, and then went on to speak about last week when he had also wanted some protection. I talked about his sore mouth last week, thinking of the hurt leg today – and I mentioned the loose tooth. "I got one pound for my tooth," he interrupted in a lively tone. "Did you?" I replied and added: "You were pleased that I remembered about your tooth and feel friendlier when you know I have remembered you. Perhaps needing to wrap yourself up today was linked with feeling hurt?" He emerged, and with great serious-ness rolled up the pillow inside the rug, using the whole floor to make a neat package which he then placed in his table-corner.

Next he looked around the room appraisingly. He fetched some water for the plants from the sink using the watering can. First, he gently sprinkled the spider plant on top of the tall cupboard, delicately removing a couple of dead leaves. "Where is the bin?" he asked and added, "It's not growing; there aren't any little ones yet." Then he moved to the plant on the window sill. "Do you water the plants?" he asked me, in a friendly tone of voice. I spoke of his ques-tions about whether I keep in mind the things that are important to him from week to week and whether I know how to look after growing things and provide what they need. In a serious tone, he said that I should take the plants out of the room when other chil-dren come in here; a younger child might pull bits off. I spoke about his doubt about allowing his different feelings to be in the room together, going on to talk to him about how the younger, wild, and angry little Tim who has often wanted to attack me, my plants, and my room, is feared by the more thoughtful Tim here just now who would like the plants and himself to grow.

Again, Tim scanned the room with careful attention. He fetched his drawing book and pencil and settled down in a corner to sketch the watering can, which he positioned with the utmost care as if he were an artist in his studio, setting up a still life. I sat on the couch and after a while spoke of his uncertainty about how close he wanted me to be today. Usually he puts a chair for me just by him, but today his mixed feelings made that seem impossible. I linked this to the upset of last week's delayed start, and his uncertainty about whether I am to be trusted. He looked up as if light were suddenly dawning, and rearranged the room to put my chair in its usual place. Then he said, "You can sit there if you want." I spoke of his not being sure if he dare tell me that this is what he wants when he is not sure if I want to be with him; when I wasn't there at the right time last week, he felt it was evidence that I did not want him.

I moved to sit by him and look at his drawing. After a few minutes he realised this altered the light and shade on the paper, and asked me to move again, showing me the light problem that was altering his composition. I moved away to re-create the original situation. He asked if he could show the picture to his father at the end of the session. I said that we would keep that in mind and think about what it meant today. I suggested that he was wanting to find a father part of me who would see that Tim is learning from me and would recognise what he feels is a good and hard-working aspect of himself. As he carried on drawing, I talked about how interested he was in light and shade today, perhaps wondering if his own light and dark feelings towards me might be able to connect up. He responded by looking behind the desk to his right, which is a very dark part of the room, particularly so on this occasion because of the bright sunshine outside. I said he now felt interested in looking into the darker places. He mouthed into the dark space "Hello, hello," and asked if I heard the echo. I spoke of his wish that I listen to a "baby" Tim that wants to explore inside himself and me.

Just as he was preoccupied with this game, he became aware of sirens outside in the road. "What's that?" he asked. I wondered what he imagined. "Murder . . . there's been an accident, someone's hurt . . . fire . . . there's a cat on a roof . . . someone's threatening to commit suicide." Then he made another reference to a fire, someone being hurt, and the ambulance getting there in time, as if recalling something he knew about. This was particularly poignant since I knew that his younger sibling had in fact died in a fire and that this had been the trigger for his being removed from his mother's care. I said Tim was thinking that today the emergency services, which he wants me to have ready for many disasters between us, might be getting there in time with the right intervention, the right ideas. Last week, when I was late, he had felt that a catastrophe had taken

171

place – he was afraid I was hurt or dead, and afraid that he would be left without help, as he had worried when Mrs D was ill and had to stop her work with him. Today he felt more hopeful that he could get a message to me about his worries about himself and me; he felt I understood how frightened he was, like a cat stranded on a roof. This made him feel that a rescue might be possible and a disaster need not happen.

He began to curl up under the little table, making a bigger space by propping the table up on one set of legs. "It's nice under here," he said with satisfaction. I said he felt he had been able to settle down with me today, and that it was like finding a safe home. Then gradually the atmosphere changed – perhaps as he noticed the evidence of some paint marks he had previously made under the table. He began to pull at the desk drawers. I said he was now wanting to poke inside all my space and find out about what did not belong to him. "Where is the phone?" he asked angrily. I said he was full of questions today about me and my room and the other people I was connected with, and was remembering the phone that used to be here. I reminded him that he knew that I had removed it because it had been too upsetting for him and too interfering to our work.

He then asked for his paints and a little water. I remarked on his wanting me to keep firmly in mind how risky things often are here, remembering so many struggles over dirty water which he loved to squirt around the room. Tim said he would be very careful, and asked for just a little water in the pot. Lying on his back, he started to dab black paint on the underside of the table. I wondered whether he could tell me about what he was doing. "All black," he said, "so no-one else can use it." As he painted I talked about Tim wanting to take over all the space here, to fill my mind up completely with him; I linked this to last week when he had felt cheated, and wanted to cover me with his spit. He went on painting very carefully underneath the table. I reminded him about his idea that if other children came in here they would want to spoil me and all my things, as he had told me earlier when he said that a little child might pull off the leaves of my plant. The other children he had in mind seemed to be like the attacking, greedy, and possessive parts of himself. I talked about how much he wished to make me into a Mrs Rustin with a label on saying "Keep out" to all the other children. "It's not only the children," he said quietly. I said this was important, he was correcting me, and explaining that he could not bear to think of anyone

172

else being with me, children or grown-ups (and at this moment I thought with pain of his mother's life as a prostitute). "I'm doing well, aren't I?" he said, in a reflective tone.

As he painted with notable care he suddenly said, "Has anyone died in the Tavi?" I asked if he could tell me any more about this question. He could only repeat it. I then said I had two ideas I wanted to share with him. Last week he had felt very afraid that I had died, but he had also been afraid that he had died in my mind, and that I had forgotten him or no longer cared about him. For little Tim this felt like my letting him die or even killing him. Now we were near the end of our session today and he was again feeling worried about whether I would be keeping him alive in my mind until next week and whether he would be able to remember me. I suggested that when it was time for our session to end he felt confused about whether I was sending him away because we had done our work for today and he could feel ready to go or whether I was throwing him out in a cruel way, as he had felt last week. We spent the last few minutes clearing up together. Tim was obviously quite anxious about his mother telling him off about the paint water that had got on to his clothes, and he picked up his sketchbook to show his father the drawing he had done in the waiting room. I thought this was to reassure himself, as his drawing would be appreciated.

Discussion

This session seemed to me to herald the possibility that links can be sustained for long enough for some modification in Tim's severely split relationship to his internal mother to take place. The acutely breathless, volatile, and edgy atmosphere of many prior sessions gives way here to some sense of rhythm, to my having enough time to say things and his having time to listen. I knew that something important had happened when we entered the room *together*. The dimension of time (Canham, 1999) was present in his mind – he wondered if I watered the plants in-between times and, in the news about his tooth money, told me something that linked both last week and this, and his external world with the therapy world. This contrasted with his usually acutely anxious desire to seal off the mayhem of the consulting room and our time together from the rather charming boy he showed himself to be in the waiting room, where he was a great favourite of the receptionists.

Once the space of the week between sessions was present for him, so were the other children who came to see me, and indeed not only children, as he himself remarked. I was perceived not as someone he must master and control because I was an unwilling and untrustworthy slave but as someone who could be asked for something and who would not be offended if the most important thing for him was not always myself – it could be that the drawing, which linked him with his daddy, was what provided something solid to hold on to at the point of separation.

The technical question he posed for me rather relentlessly was what I could afford to risk. Black paint all over the floor, and on me, for example. The important point, I think, was that I was not to know and had to endure the pain of taking the risk. If I imposed too many limits, I implied no trust at all in his potential for responsible behaviour, but I had to live with this knowledge of his capacity for sadistic delight in cynical trickery, alongside the appreciation of being understood and finding meaning.

Broader reflections

The clinical process with Tim highlights some central Kleinian and post-Kleinian concepts, which have proved particularly relevant to work with abused and deprived children. Klein's (1936) originality in describing the intense neediness of the infant for responsive maternal care was to see that the infant's anxieties arose not only from the fact of initial total dependence but also from the urgent pressure to be relieved of the terror aroused by his own overwhelming impulses. She conceptualised the baby's love and hate as rooted in the life and death instincts with which the infant is confronted from the start of life. The role of the mother can then be understood as not only the provision of physical care for the baby to ensure survival and growth, but also of psychological receptivity to modify his fears of abandonment. Bion's development of a theory of the growth of mind that showed the process of preverbal communication between infant and mother taking place through the mechanism of projective identification, maternal reverie, and understanding elaborated Klein's description of the object-relatedness of the baby from birth onwards.

Tim's sensitivity to any feelings of loss of safety is more than understandable from the point of view of his early experience.

174

Frequent brief episodes of being cared for by unknown people when his mother could not cope, a preoccupied mother with no stable home and abusive partners, the death of a sibling, permanent loss of mother's care and subsequent loss of a foster-mother when placed for adoption, all added to by the loss of his first therapist, exposed him to a repeated experience of existential threat. The absence of a reliable external parental figure meant that his internal world was peopled by figures he suspected and could not trust. The volatility in his relationship with me was, however, as became clear, due not only to his vulnerability to believing me to be another abandoning maternal figure but also to the unpredictable upsurges of violent mistrust and hatred that threatened him with having nowhere to project his aggression. If I was not there, could he survive? "Has anyone died in the Tavistock?" he asked, and I think at depth this question referred to his anxiety about both his lost internal maternal object and his own endangered healthy self. The frightening black hole of his lost tooth and his marked sense of painful bodily vulnerability both express the visceral quality of a very early fear of loss of life, of absence of protection from deathly anxieties. Bick's description of early infantile states (Bick, 1964, 1968) and Tustin's later work on this theme (Tustin, 1981) have become classics for child psychotherapists in much of their work with severely disturbed children.

The growth of capacities for observation, reflection, and memory is what can modify the profound insecurity of the infant. The child who has had many changes of primary carer early in life has, however, a particular area of loss with respect to memory. The story of his early life is not known to the parents who are bringing him up. In my work with Tim, I thought my giving him evidence of my capacity to recall details from earlier sessions was very important to him. It provided him with an experience of my having a functioning memory that could store what was relevant and draw on it. In later work with him, it was his growing ability to distinguish past, present, and an imagined future, that seemed to usher in his readiness to work towards ending his therapy.

A second critical issue was of course the question of whether things could be put right. What balanced Klein's deep concern with the distinctive forces in mental life was not only her attention to the balance of love and hate in the personality but also her discovery of the impulse to repair. In the early months of work with Tim it was precisely the absence of any sense of concern about the impact of his ruthless behaviour that was most disturbing to me. This echoed what greatly upset his parents, who feared that his habitual lying and complete refusal to acknowledge any fault presaged a psychopathic delinquent future. It was, therefore, of great significance when reparative and creative behaviour emerged (Segal, 1957). His willingness to tackle clearing up the pornographic mess he had made in daubing my wall opened up the possibility of the creative use of art materials to explore internal and external reality.

His artistic expansiveness also represented oedipal development. The dominant configuration at the start was one in which parental intercourse was represented as continuous, violent, ugly, and perverse, something inflicted on the child in order to torment him with feelings of exclusion, powerlessness, and humiliation. At the start in the countertransference, one of my striking experiences was the loneliness I felt, not only the loneliness of the neglected infant that Tim often projected on to me, but also the loneliness of having no adult to turn to in my own mind. No doubt this had something to do with my feeling echoes of his mother's unsupported circumstances in his first two years, but I also saw it as a broken oedipal link in which I as mother could find no father during the sessions. Sometimes I found myself needing to talk to a colleague afterwards to recover a sense of reality and my awareness of potential support. The oedipal triangle was, therefore, marked by its frequent absence (O'Shaughnessy, 1989). When Tim began to draw – and also when he could use paper to write, in the form of messages, thoughts that were too difficult to say out loud – mental space seemed present in a new way. Symbolic expression went hand in hand with new possibilities with respect to the oedipal triangle. Tim and father could have a link of which I was the observer, as described by Britton (1989) and at the same time I could find my mind at work freely, able to be in intercourse with my psychoanalytic intuition and intellectual resources afresh.

What is unavoidable when there is serious early abuse and neglect as well as loss is that the therapist is going to have to survive being badly treated and feeling neglected over a long period. Only if the child can feel that she has really taken in what it means to count for nothing, to face much cruelty, and to believe one is alone in the world is there going to be the possibility of his discovery of a mind that can take the measure of his experience and not throw it back

176

at him. To do this work, the psychoanalytic concepts I have mentioned were a vital resource. Also needed is an institution able to acknowledge the clinical necessities of adequate time for such work, team support, and recognition of an inevitable degree of disruption of the physical environment as well as of the state of mind of the therapist. However, these are the children likely to be a huge cost to themselves, their families, and the wider society in future years if left without therapeutic help. It is a remarkable thing that psychoanalysis has provided us with theories that make it possible to intervene and to make a difference, and it is vital that such work should be protected in the future.

Note

1 An earlier version of this paper was published in 2001 as 'The Therapist with Her Back against the Wall', *Journal of Child Psychotherapy*, 27 (3): 273–284.

WHERE IS THE PAIN?

Body, mind, and family culture (2005)

In the psychoanalytic psychotherapy of a boy who seems most of the time to feel himself likely to be misunderstood, I have found myself thinking about the connection between the painful absence of reciprocity between him and his parental figures and also about the nature of the internal worlds of his parents and of their way of relating to each other. Everyone in this family of three is in pain, but there is little capacity to recognize each other's distress.

I shall begin by referring to the model developed by Harris and Meltzer (1976, 1986) about family patterns. The core parental task, they suggest, is the containment of the mental pain associated with growth and development. They described family functioning as influenced by pairs of polarities which are in a state of dynamic flux:

- Generating love v promulgating hate
- Promoting hope v sowing despair
- Containing depressive pain v emanating persecutory anxiety
- Thinking v creating confusion

It will be obvious that the balance of projective and introjective tendencies is part of this model. The varieties of family relationship they could differentiate using this theory they named as 'couple families', with a subgroup of this category, the 'Doll's House family', 'matriarchal' or 'patriarchal' families, 'gang' families, 'reversed' families and 'basic assumption' families.

The family of my patient reminded me of the description of the Doll's House family. Meltzer and Harris suggested that this structure

DOI: 10.4324/9781003325543-15

is a consequence of parents who have been unable to identify with the adolescent community as they grew up and have thus continued in a kind of latency position with respect to their own parents – needing to fulfil parental expectations, tending to espouse conformity, to lack courage, independent judgement and imagination. The wider community is likely to be partially avoided, while its authority figures are held in awe, though secretly denigrated. The characteristic parental injunction to be 'good' children lends itself to a sense of moral superiority, and the overriding desire is to achieve and hold on to security. Illness, economic setbacks and any obvious difficulties in the children's development are consequently sources of panic. In the more intimate area of family life, the secretiveness which is characteristic of the family's relationship to the wider community also appears in the family's relationships, and open emotionality and awareness of sexuality is avoided. The place of bodily experience in family life is thus doubly compromised – there is deep anxiety both about sexuality and about any illness. Somatization of mental pain tends to occur due to the failure of relational development.

This creates a setting in which the baby who has a capacity for passionate engagement is faced with painful or incomprehensible frustration, in which the hope of reciprocity is likely to be replaced by the experience of misfit and misunderstanding. One risk in this impasse is that the blocked impulses of love turn to hatred and violence. If the child persists in attempting to communicate despite the discouragement of an impervious object, there is still a possibility of contact being made, for the child to find somewhere to lodge the longing for recognition and for the overwhelming nature of the feelings evoked by the encounter with parental figures to be contained. However, if despair takes over, deterioration sets in because the desire for communication is atrophied. Indeed, the desire for life itself may be undermined. My patient, following a particularly horrendous scene at home, wrote a note for his parents in which he said he did not deserve to live and that he wished to be buried with his teddy and his cowboy hat. The parents brought this note to the clinic to convey their desperation, but seemed not to be able to give any meaning to his references to his beloved teddy or to his cowboy hat. I remember thinking that the agony of failed understanding was poignantly conveyed in this episode. The parent workers have the painful and repeated experience that if they explore the possible symbolic significance of any of Adam's behaviour, to try and expand the parents' understanding of their son, they are usually rubbished and mocked for their interest in the idea of behaviour having any meaning. A relationship between parents which interferes with the primary mother-child link, which is the case in my patient's family, can provoke dangerous levels of rage and potential violence.

Clinical material

My patient, Adam, is now nine years old. I have seen him for 18 months, initially in once weekly psychotherapy, which was then increased to twice a week. His parents are seen weekly by a couple of colleagues, a rather unusual arrangement which reflects the clinic's assessment that only very regular input and the resilience of a therapeutic couple had any chance of shifting the deadly state of affairs in the family. Adam was adopted at birth from abroad. We do not know why the couple were unable to conceive since they do not easily share information of this personal kind, but a picture of their family backgrounds has begun to emerge. Mother's mother died when she was very young. Father's family is deeply shadowed by holocaust losses in the previous generation which we came to know about through Adam's communications to me, and not from Father himself. They are practising but not orthodox Jews.

When I first met the parents, I had been warned to expect a difficult encounter. They had sought and received help from various local services of which they were extremely contemptuous, and had now approached what they called the 'experts', that is the specialist Adoption team at the Tavistock Clinic. The consultant psychiatrist and senior social worker who initially met the family were deeply alarmed – they felt that Adam was at serious risk since, when enraged, he would assault his mother and then run off into the road. They found the parents unable to listen to Adam, themselves or the clinicians. Mother and Father arrived armed with notebooks which contained details of all Adam's terrible behaviour which they wished to recount, and held their pens poised when the clinicians spoke, to record whatever was said, which they hoped would be the expert advice and instruction they craved. In the clinical team discussion, it was decided that an experienced child psychotherapist must assess Adam, since Father's tendency to demolish what others say was likely to be stirred up by the assessment process. I dealt with this potential threat by being rather firm in what I would offer – an individual assessment followed by a further consultation with the parents to discuss my recommendations. Having started out with the probable intention of referring the boy to a child psychotherapy trainee for intensive treatment, I ended up feeling that therapeutic discontinuity was an impossible course of action, and that I would have to see him myself even though this meant less intensive treatment, due to my own limited availability.

Working with Adam always feels that one may at any moment face a breakdown in connection. There are never sessions in which I can afford to relax my watchfulness. This is both because of his great attraction to deceiving me, to lulling me into a false confidence that we are in an honest interchange, when he is in fact trying to trick me about something, and because of the impulsiveness and violence of his behaviour when we are in conflict. He loves to taunt me with the threat of an unmanageable flood, a broken window, smashed furniture or one or other of us getting injured. As he plays quite wildly, recreating scenes of war, terrorism and catastrophe, he often sustains minor tumbles which he seems to experience as serious hurts, maybe even broken limbs, his moans can imply. He is hugely excited by the idea that he can make me feel terror, lose hope or start hating him. At the same time, if I miss the evidence of his positive attachment to me and to his therapy which he often invites me to do by filling me with anxiety and apprehension, I am aware of repeating in the transference relationship his experience of being unheld and unwanted. I have become alert to the idea that moments of progress occur particularly when there is a palpable nearness to the edge in the atmosphere of the session. If it can be survived – acknowledged and contained but not amplified – something tends to take place in which more straightforward ways of relating are represented, and which also has the transformative quality of introducing what I experience as an aesthetic dimension. I will give two examples of this.

The first occurred following a session in which Adam had been murderously angry with me when I insisted that the drawing he had done, a tracing of a war-plane and missiles from a book he brought to the session (typical of his intense preoccupation with war), must stay with me. I had spoken of the value of the things done in the room for our work together – they belonged to both of us. The next time he arrived looking very grim. He angrily emptied his box of toys all over the floor, but then extracted particular things from the chaos, while pretending that he had successfully tricked me about his paper supplies and thus extracted more. I felt sure he was trying to get me into a negative, suspicious state of mind. He sat down with a sheet of fresh paper and said he wanted a sharp knife to score some shapes. This might have been a point of breakdown, but he realized with some simple observations from me about what I had provided for him that he could use the scissors and also the sharp edge of the ruler he had previously broken in rage. He cut out three shapes, somewhat like triangles, asking (unusually) for some help from me in doing this. These he placed on top of a second sheet making them touch each other. Then he made a border, and stuck it down with glue. Next he carefully coloured in the shapes in a kind of patch-work of bright colours – he usually uses only black, so colour has always been a precious indication of the emergence of warmth. He made a decorative border which he called 'the frame'.

I spoke to him about three shapes joining in his picture – might this be like three people joining to make a family? How complicated it was to wait and see how they might fit together as he had wanted me to wait to see how his picture turned out. Was this also like the two of us here working at how things might be joined up inside Adam, and how we could join up all the sharp and angry feelings with some more patient and friendly ones? Today he perhaps felt this was rather an important idea. Adam gave me his creation at the end of the session asking me to keep it safe. It was clear he wanted it kept separate from the jumble in his box in which most of his drawings are at risk of destruction when he is full of fury.

In this session, I believe we can see the creative impulse in Adam emerge and develop, protected by splitting off into me the paranoid, spoiling part of himself. Later, as he becomes aware that I have contained the destructive suspicion, he can make contact with a helping-me and there is a moving experience of us working as an analytic couple. It is articulated in his beautiful and interesting artefact.

In the second example, I was almost broken by the violence of his projections, and had to recover myself before his eyes. This hap-pened following a difficult end to the previous session in which he had tried to 'kill' my plants, as he put it, by secretly dousing them in hot water, pretending that it was cold and that he was taking care of them. When I intervened, he triumphantly broke the string of my window blind. It seemed clear that I was to be left miserable, hav-ing witnessed his joy in destruction. At the beginning of the next session, he told me about the March Hare in Alice in Wonderland who says 'I'm late . . . ' and muddles up Easter and Christmas. As this session preceded a Bank Holiday one session break, I said he was feeling that time got all muddled up when a session was cancelled – perhaps it was hard to remember that we would meet again next Wednesday as usual. I distinguished the big boy Adam who can remember and the very small boy Adam who can't sort it out and feels that everything gets mixed up. He took a large lump of plasticine out of his box and began a catching game with me as if it were a ball. Then suddenly the plasticine ball became a weapon hurled at me with intent to hurt and at the window with intent to smash it. After an undignified struggle, with his lifting a chair to throw at me, I said that he was not allowed to hurt me or damage the room seriously and that if he continued I would have to stop the session to give him some time to cool off in the waiting room. (I had never actually done this at this point.) He hurled a chair at me, and I said that I would now take him back to the waiting room for five minutes. He resisted with all his strength and, close to tears, was clearly in the grip of a terrible panic. Acknowledging that I was angry because he had hurt me, I said 'Let's try and find another way to sort things out'. I returned to my chair and he sheltered in the far corner. I described what had happened, and spoke about how maddened he was by the missing session and how he had needed me to understand that.

He began to build a 'safe house' using all the available furniture. The blanket and cushions were crucial elements, making me aware of his need for something soft, receptive and protective to recover from the acting-out he had evoked from me. He asked for my help in constructing the roof of the house (from the couch-mattress). As he rested inside, peeping through gaps and asking every few moments if I could see him, I spoke about how he felt I had not understood that he felt hurt and angry when he did not see me – in his mind I became a going-away, forgetting Mrs Rustin. He had felt he had to hurt me to get me to understand how hurt he was. 'I didn't hurt you very badly' he said. I agreed, and said it was really important for us to understand what goes so wrong when he feels upset. He fetched a pen and secretly wrote on the wall 'Adam [heart shape] Megan', boasting that the writing would not come off, but told me what he had written when I asked. I said he wanted me to know he was a boy who can love people and he wanted to let me know that because he was afraid of how much he sometimes hates me and how afraid he is that he can make me hate him. Not coming next Monday makes him afraid he will be homesick for me and worried that he's lost me inside himself. I added that he wanted to leave his name on my wall to force me to remember him and to hold on to his place in my mind over the gap. Later in the session, as I could feel him calm down, he spontaneously got water from the sink and cleaned off the writing very carefully. At the end, we put the room to rights together.

Reflecting on this session, I saw that a central feature was the projection of humiliation, which I had failed to contain in my initial retreat to behavioural sanctions. The split second moment at which the plasticine ball became a weapon felt like a blow to my willingness to trust – an exploitation of my foolish innocence. I responded with a counter-attack but I quickly realized how humiliated he would be in front of his mother if I carried out my threat. In retrospect, I saw in my mind's eye the infant poised between the mother who had just given birth and the one he was being handed to. Cruelty, confusion, hurt and humiliation were displacing a potentially tender encounter. In the countertransference experience, I became an unrecognisably distorted and ugly version of myself – failing to understand, using adult power to assert my will, completely out of contact with an internal paternal presence which could help me to be aware of my adult capacity for thought and in touch with my patient's littleness and vulnerability. Only when I got back to my chair could I re-establish a psychoanalytic attitude in myself and start to make sense of things. These terrible moments of being overwhelmed by the impact of a patient's projections are suffused with shame. Recovering a sense of perspective, of course, involved my being able to see myself in a more kindly light – to clean up the mess I had made of things, one might say, in a non-persecuted way, which I think was echoed by Adam's later washing the wall he had written on, which he did quietly and thoroughly, and without fuss. All this underlined the links between decency (ethical behaviour) and images of coherence, tenderness and beauty on the one hand and ruthlessness (the denial of all concern) and chaos, imperviousness and ugliness on the other. In fact it is striking that Adam is a child who can look really nice (open and eager) at one moment, and absolutely horrible and chilling at others, when viciousness has temporarily triumphed.

It is striking to me how the theory of the Doll's House family I referred to earlier (Harris and Meltzer) helps to illuminate the problems that I struggle with in my work with Adam. I have noted the collapse of the analytic couple within me during the session described and we can readily see the latency-style retreat to rules, the absence of imagination, the over-sensitivity to physical hurt and the assumed moral legitimacy of my position. But I am also interested in the role of shame, which seems to become a dominant emotion and to replace the guilt and concern which would signal the move back into an object-related position from a predominantly narcissistic one.

A recent sequence of sessions threw some further light on the centrality of shame and disappointment (Emanuel, 1984; Cregeen, 2009). Again, a missing session in prospect, due to the parental decision to cancel a session so that Adam could be at his school sports day, was the trigger. Adam spent a long time inflicting sadistic tortures on a toy owl which he has always been fascinated. He played the part of the owl ('Mr Owl') begging in a small child's voice for mercy as well as that of the torturer. Mr Owl was repeatedly held under water as well as being violently hurled around the room. I said to him that the torturing Adam could not bear the idea that Mr Owl and other children who came to see me would be in this room on Wednesday when he would miss his session. This made him so jealous that he wanted to kill off knowing about his upset feelings and pretend that he was a person without any feelings except excitement in cruelty and killing. He was trying to forget how fond he is of Mr Owl and how difficult it is not to be able to come here. He was not helped by this line of interpretation and became wilder at the sink so that I had to intervene to prevent a major flood. The violence then escalated and he kicked me repeatedly. I said I would put his shoes outside the room until the end of the session as I could not allow him to hurt me in this way and I could see he could not stop himself. He was very angry but in fact tolerated my doing this, but shortly afterwards threw a hard toy directly at my face and hurt me quite badly. I was extremely shocked and it took some moments for me to be able to think at all. Adam was ranting about how he did not care about Wednesday, that I was a stupid ugly bitch, therapy was shit and that I thought he was crap. The important thing in all this seemed to me to be that the therapist he was attacking was one he believed to be hostile and rejecting towards him and that we were dealing with the unbearable experience of primary rejection. Adam's infantile self felt perceived as a crap baby, not one worth looking after. An annihilating experience of humiliation.

The knife-edge I felt up against was indeed that my hate, panic and fear would overpower my capacity for thought and concern. Adam had momentarily succeeded in projecting so much confusion, hatred, persecution and despair that I was overwhelmed. I thought the danger almost engulfing us was that there would be a transference re-enactment of the shame and guilt of a mother who cannot care for her baby and of a baby who feels he is simply an ugly disappointment. We were thus facing the possible death of the therapy. The shame of the adoptive parents unable to conceive a child, and Adam's awareness of and cruel exploitation of this, was a further important dimension of what was being enacted. The fact that Adam has been loved and cared for to the best of his parents' abilities and that I have worked very hard to help him was at risk of obliteration in the face of this dominating internal configuration.

Containment required the internal reconstruction of my relationship to a helpful paternal presence, to re-find the penis-as-link and escape from the persecuting assertion of phallic omnipotence (Birksted-Breen, 1996). This required consultation with a supervisor, and a great deal of thought about how to create a safe setting for me and Adam through introducing some new rules and through attempting to protect him from intolerable provocations. I also decided to formally report my injury according to clinical governance regulations as a way of helping me to take what had happened seriously enough and not to become blind to the murderous impulses unleashed.

Family culture

I now want to comment on the contribution of the family culture to Adam's problems. In work with children where we may have some access to knowledge of the parents' own difficulties, we are in the unusual position of being able to think about the child's internal parental figures as understood through the transference/countertransference relationship alongside some understanding of the actual parents' internal worlds. What can be particularly painful is the recognition that the child's potential for development may not be supported by family capacities. As I noted earlier, this leaves the dangerous dynamic of toxic forms of misunderstanding potentially active in ongoing family relationships. This is an unavoidable area of risk in analytic work with children, and one has to question oneself carefully about whether the child's potential for self-understanding

186

may become adequate to protect him from destructive enactments even if the parents remain impervious to change.

In this family, when there are periods of development in Adam, and a softening in the parent/child hostilities, there is a recurrent pattern of illness emerging as a parental preoccupation. There are somewhat frail grandparents on both sides of the family, so hospital admissions and visits recurrently take over the mental space of one or both parents. Their faces become grey, burdened with anxiety, and Adam's efforts to engage them become more desperate. With his mother this usually leads to physical assaults by Adam from which she cannot protect herself. This of course fuels further anxiety about his capacity to destroy. He arrives for sessions with intense accounts of having hurt himself and hugely exaggerated claims of pain and injury. When emotional communication breaks down, pain has to become a physical reality. His excruciating anxiety about being able to be loved is enacted in hateful behaviour towards his mother which leaves them both hopeless. The relationship has been reduced to one of physical expression, and hurt bodies replace their wounded feelings as the focus.

The important point here is that clinical attention needs to attend to the loss of mental capacities for symbolization, verbal communication and thought which underlies the hurt bodies we are confronted with. 'The body speaks' we might say, if we listen to it, and when we can pick up the message, we can re-connect body and emotional experience for our patients. Meaning can then begin to emerge.

In work with children and families, this approach to somatic phenomena also involves clarifying whose pain is at the heart of the problem. In my case example, both parents and Adam were suffering though in very different ways, but very often we can have situations where one member of a family is manifesting distress, but may at depth be carrying this for someone else. This makes it enormously important not to think in terms of collections of symptoms adding up to a treatable named condition but instead of people in complex intimate relationships, internal and external, whose equilibrium is painfully disturbed. Clinical intervention has to be at both internal and external levels if long term change is to be achieved.

It is worth asking why the referral of Adam came at the point it did, as it was clear that many difficulties at home had been there from the start. One factor may have been the growth spurt, which turned him rather quickly from a little boy into quite a tall one and one whose athleticism was what he most valued in himself. He was also rather handsome when not overtaken by bad feelings, and while this might have given his parents pleasure, and indeed sometimes did, as for example in his marked success in school shows, I think it was also a threat. He did not look like them, and both he and they were preoccupied by his birth family with whom limited contact had been maintained. His energetic devotion to demanding exercise often filled much of his session time; when he felt full of muscle power, his omnipotence was fuelled, even though, as I described, this could collapse in spectacular fashion if something did not quite work out. His mother was not a frail woman but she was clearly frightened of him when he got into a rage. One could suggest that the recognition of the approach of puberty challenged her capacity to feel a competent parent, since the latency mode of functioning shared by the couple had its origin in a failure to embrace adolescent sexuality. Adam was of course alert to his parents' vulnerabilities in coping with sexual matters and was an expert at taunting his mother (and me) with humiliating dirty talk. Adoptive parents and children have a life-long task in relating to the child's original family in the mind and this has to be re-worked at each developmental stage. The Harris/Meltzer family typology I referred to earlier can of course be fruitfully seen as delineating the developmental challenges inherent in family life and therefore very useful in understanding the difficulties that parents need help with in child and adolescent services.

SECTION 4

WORKING WITH PARENTS

DIALOGUES WITH PARENTS (1998)

This chapter is an overview of an approach to work with parents practised within the multi-disciplinary teams which were for a long period the bedrock of child, adolescent and family mental health services within the NHS. In more recent years the composition of many of these teams has changed, sometimes quite radically, and the depth of work with parents now available has been diluted, often replaced by group psycho-educational interventions. I shall however describe the rich possibilities that psychoanalytically trained therapists can offer to support parents troubled by their children's difficulties. These forms of work remain relevant and are to be found in the varied settings where child psychotherapy is available and are also the basis for much private practice.

History of work with parents within child guidance

Perhaps it would be useful to start with some historical background. The early generations of child psychotherapists could rely on close working partnerships with experienced social workers (Harris, 1968). The post-war Child Guidance Clinics were fortunate in their genuine multidisciplinary ethos and particularly in their social workers, who usually had a commitment to a psychoanalytically based understanding of human development and family relationships. Much of Winnicott's writing about his hospital work is imbued with his sense of the multidisciplinary teams within which his creative potential developed and standards of good practice were established. This was a very particular culture of care.

DOI: 10.4324/9781003325543-17

The child cases I took on during my training and in the early years after qualification were often supported either by long-term work with the mother of the referred child or by work with the couple, where the focus might be on the couple's relationship. Psychiatric social workers had the skill of bearing the actual child in mind while finding ways to address the anxieties of parents (Shuttleworth, 1982). Their work tended to be on the borderline of case work (by this I mean work intended to support parental functioning) and psychotherapy. Proper use was made of the transference as a source of evidence of emotional conflicts, but it was rather rarely used explicitly. However, during this period there was a sea-change going on in the training and professional framework of social work, which was eroding such forms of practice. By the late 1970s, interest in internal aspects of relationship difficulties had waned and family therapy was the dominant therapeutic tool of interest to social workers. Child psychotherapists had to rethink how to approach work with parents.

The approach of child psychotherapists

This situation led to many of us seeing the way forward as one in which we would need to be able to support each other's cases. It was frequently noted that, unless long-term work with parents was provided, the child's therapy was at risk of interruption, irregular attendance and so on. Who better to provide the necessary input than one of our own colleagues? However, this development raised important questions of technique. We were very carefully trained in working within the psychoanalytic model of observation of transference and countertransference phenomena, and the interpretation of unconscious material, with insight as a primary goal of the work, but this kind of approach was by no means always appropriate or acceptable to parents. So we had to learn to use our observations of underlying patterns of object relations in different ways. We also found ourselves exposed to shaky marriages, borderline personalities, the risk of adult psychotic breakdown, perverse family structures and so on, and all of these, while they could be approached coherently on the basis of the training in work with children and adolescents, also took us into new territory. I do not think we have fully resolved the consequences of this either in terms of training or in thinking deeply enough about the clinical issues. Seminars in work with parents are a requirement in the Tavistock training, but often this work can be very difficult indeed. Does the absence of an expectation of individual supervision reduce the attention given to this work and its status? Is the work done of an adequate quality? Perhaps our anxieties on this score are one source of the tendency for child psychotherapists to go on to train as adult therapists or analysts. There are often excellent reasons for people seeking this extension of their professional capacities, but possibly some of the pressure to seek further training is a consequence of our not having solved the problem of how to train for the component of adult work within any child psychotherapist's practice.

A possible model

In reviewing the range of work undertaken with parents, I have come to think about four main categories. At one end of the spectrum are cases where gaining the support of parents to protect and sustain the child's therapy is the prime aim. The second group is where parents are looking for support in their parental functioning. The development of brief work with the parents of babies and small children is a specialization within this category (Daws, 1989; Miller, 1992). This group includes parents who feel they cannot make sense of a child's behaviour and relationships and who seek a better understanding of their children's problems, and parents who are struggling to cope with very difficult life circumstances – family illness, economic stress, disability, bereavement and so on. These parents either see themselves as working in partnership with the professionals or feel in need of help themselves, but with the focus clearly on their role as parents. The third group is where the explicit aim of the work is change in family functioning, and this has been agreed by the parents as part of the treatment as a whole. There are different styles of work which may be appropriate, including marital therapy, individual work with a focus on the intra-family relationships or family therapy as such. At the other end of the spectrum is individual psychotherapy for one or indeed both parents, to which the parents have committed themselves as patients in their own right, even if the issues which have brought them into contact with psychotherapists have started off as concern for a child. Both the therapies aimed at change within the family and psychoanalytic psychotherapy can function either alongside treatment of a child or on their own. I fully realize that these categories are schematic and that clinical cases often face us with work that veers between one and another type of work, but I think it may be useful nonetheless to have the broad range subdivided. Sometimes the move from one position to another on this spectrum needs not only to be grasped by ourselves but also rendered explicit to patients. It is a bit like the transition from assessment into ongoing therapy. If work in progress makes it clear that a different aim from that originally intended is appropriate, signalling this can both give us real consent for a change in technique and enable us to free ourselves from confusion about what we are responsible for. My examples will address some of these points further.

First clinical example

Let me take first the support of a child's treatment. A recent example comes vividly to mind. An eight-year-old boy was about to begin three times a week treatment. His evangelical Christian parents are separated. Both are closely involved with their two children. The boy had previously attended a one-year children's group therapy, and his mother had joined a parallel parental group of which she spoke with warmth. She then requested individual help for herself and had been offered weekly sessions. Father, however, needed to be catered for in addition. The parents' relationship is stormy, full of writs and injunctions as well as real efforts to share out the care of the children. Mr A has a tendency to manic-depressive episodes and has made a serious suicidal attempt. He is under the care of a psychiatrist and also has had some counselling arranged as part of his psychiatric care. He has shown himself to be very touchy indeed about being treated as of equal importance to his wife in relation to his son. Faxes to the chief executive with complaints about clinic staff are part of the fat file which I inherited at the point when one of my tutees was to take on the boy's therapy. What should we offer this father? Seeing the potential for trouble, I decided that a very clearcut approach would be best. I offered Mr A an initial meeting in my role as Case Consultant – this is the title given at the Tavistock to the clinical manager of a case. In this I negotiated that I would be seeing him together with his son's therapist (a young man for whom this was a first intensive case) each term, to review the progress of the psychotherapy. If anything arose in between these meetings, Mr A was invited to get in contact with me. Despite the alarming tone of the threats he uttered in his initial meeting with me – he announced he would not hesitate to consult his lawyer or to complain to all relevant authorities if he felt in any way left out of any decisions about his son's treatment, or indeed mistreated in any other way – Mr A has in fact been supportive of the boy's therapy overall, and taken a share in bringing him to sessions.

My feeling was that a number of factors had to be taken into account: first, this father needed to feel taken seriously as having parental responsibility and not dismissed as mentally ill; second, he needed the clinic to provide an absolutely clear account of who was responsible for what, particularly since the prior management of the case had been rather confused; third, the responsibility for containing Mr A had to lie with a senior member of staff who had the confidence to stand up to potential bullying and who would be seen as having authority both by the family and by the members of the clinical team. As psychotherapists we usually veer away from taking an authoritative stance, but I think there are circumstances where the assertion of professional authority is appropriate, when it is based on knowledge and a willingness to take responsibility. This can be the best containment of an unstable parent.

Parents who seek support

Now let us look at work with parents who are openly seeking support. I would like to refer to two contrasting cases, both concerning the parents of autistic children. It should be mentioned that this group of parents is one with special needs, both because of the complexity of the network of services with which their child is likely to be involved and because of the peculiar loneliness often felt within these families (Klauber, 1998). Their children are so difficult to understand and to integrate into social life. One helpful approach tried out by Sue Reid and Trudy Klauber (Reid, 1999b) was the establishment of a group for these parents, meeting once a term or so for an extended evening meeting, when some of their shared concerns could be discussed. Parents felt helped by each other in coping with family and community issues. This group was in addition to the regular work undertaken with them on a case basis.

To undertake supportive work with parents, two possible models can be considered. The first is when the child's therapist also works with the parents. This can be seen as an extension of the termly review meetings, and is appropriate when the parents seem very reluctant to see anyone else. It may of course also be the only option available in the context of limited resources. When the referred child is psychotic or autistic, there can be good reasons for parents wishing to maintain a close contact with the child's therapist. He or she is often the person most able to help them understand the very puzzling character of their child's behaviour, and, if some understanding of bizarre rituals or explosive tantrums can be achieved, it is easier for parents to sort out their response (Tischler, 1979).

Second clinical example

In my work with a psychotic girl whom I saw for psychotherapy for nine years, from age 13 to 22, I found that the work with her parents, which I had taken on reluctantly, was in fact fruitful, although I had started out by wishing that they would accept my offer to find them a colleague who would see them regularly. As they gained confidence in my commitment to working with this very ill girl, saw that I could make some sense of her behaviour and communications, and would take seriously how immensely burdensome her illness was to all the other members of the family, they began to give up some of their defensiveness. Mother in particular had told a tale of extensive prior contact with professionals by whom she felt blamed for Holly's autism; in fact in the early years she had been told that she was the one who needed psychiatric treatment, as it was her anxiety not anything in her child which was the problem. Her conviction that I recognized the agonies that Holly endured, and also appreciated how painful it was to be close to her and feel responsibility for her, was the basis of increasing trust in me.

I met these parents once or sometimes twice each term throughout Holly's treatment. Occasionally, these meetings also included, at the parents' request, another professional with responsibility for an aspect of Holly's life. For example, when a local authority social worker became involved in relation to possible residential placement when Holly was 18, she joined us, and later, when Holly moved to live in the community, the nun in charge of the institution she joined, a woman with immense good sense and a capacity to enjoy the good qualities of damaged young people, also came from time to time. The parents saw me as Holly's interpreter on these occasions, with the task of making sure that other professionals had a proper grasp of what sort of person she was. They also valued my willingness to face and to speak up for the realities – they often felt subjected to pressures to agree to what they felt was against Holly's interests, in particular, to deny the extent of her pain and her illness and to adopt a spurious cheerfulness about her future.

In the work with the parents themselves, there were four major areas where useful work was done, and one where I felt defeated. This last was in my efforts to create space for consideration of Holly's younger sister, for whom I felt concerned, but I never succeeded in this. The first matter we tackled was to explore what could be done about Holly's ruthless splitting of the parents. She rejected her mother systematically and indeed all things female, while idealizing her father, who was an art teacher. She spent hours entrancing him with what he saw initially as remarkable creativity. This consisted mostly in model-making, at which she was deft, the models being delusional penises (lighthouses, windmills, etc.) which she made by the dozen. These were felt by her to support her absolute denial of her own femininity. Her hatred and mistrust of her mother was painfully recognized by Mother as in part a response to Mother's hatred of her in her early years. This mother's sense of rejection, faced with an autistic baby, combined disastrously with fear rooted in the history of mental illness in her family of origin to create a pool of hatred which she knew she had been unable to contain. But the vengefulness of Holly's refusal to recognize the loving and devoted side of her mother needed a change of stance from father: he had to stand up to her distortions, and to challenge his own narcissistic pleasure in being the preferred parent. My involvement in the overall care of Holly resurrected respect for the maternal role, allowed Mother to regain some sense of her importance to Holly, and Father to give back to her some of his ill-gotten gains and to share with her the heaviness of the task of confronting Holly at times. The reversal of roles had been at the expense of Mother's capacity for tenderness and of his capacity for firmness.

A second focus was how Holly might be shifted from her defensive obsessional rituals. Over the years, as they felt more confidence in me, they were able to turn to me for help in gathering courage to assert themselves against her deadening demand for sameness. They ultimately rebelled against the tyranny of having to go on the same bus ride, have the same meals on predictable days of the week and answer the same questions for the thousandth time. Their conversations with each other and me enabled them to see that Holly's belief that she would fall to pieces if her will was challenged was unreal. Her tantrums had been so explosive and so overwhelming to them that they had boxed themselves into a shared phantasy about Holly's need to be treated as tenderly as an egg, as though her identity was a shell always at risk of shattering. Related to this process of becoming empowered as parents and escaping from Holly's rigid control was their struggle to assert themselves against the maternal grandmother who had maintained a malignant idealization of Holly, which overlooked her capacity to devastate others' lives as well as her own. Mother found in me an ally, to sustain her against the denigratory and envy-loaded projections of her own mother and against her daughter's projections of despair, meaninglessness and unending guilt. Discussing the details of Holly's peculiar preoccupations sometimes enabled them to find meaning in what had become impossible for them to think about, because it seemed so strangely impenetrable. They became more able to distinguish between what had valuable meaning and was worth listening to and pondering and what was fundamentally an attack on meaningfulness and required parental limit-setting. Family life had been shaped by an anxiously compliant respect for Holly's problems which needed to come into question. For example, when she asked for the hundredth time for reassurance that she would not have to share a room or a bed with her sister on the family holiday, was it constructive to answer as if this was a reasonable question or was it reasonable to express irritation and refuse to go along with her claim not to know what had already been carefully explained to her?

A third important area was in helping them to make steps towards some separation. Holly had had a catastrophic early separation from home. When she was four, she had been placed in a psychiatric hospital at a distance from home for almost a year, spending only weekends with her family. Mother understood deeply that this had been severely traumatic for Holly. In fact ultimately Mother had refused to take her back because the weekly separations had been so unbearably painful. Her guilt about this enforced early separation made any move towards thinking of Holly leaving home very difficult. This arose first in discussion of schooling. When I first met her, Holly was going to a local school for learning disabled children. This was profoundly unsuitable – she was driving the teachers crazy with her loud psychotic chatter throughout the day and she was being actively abused by other children in the playground, who were frightened of her madness and dealt with this by exploiting and degrading her. A change of school meant a long journey, and ultimately a weekly boarding arrangement, with weekends at home. Holly and Mother shared a sense of impending catastrophe about this: Mother felt she would never be forgiven for a second separation and Holly believed she was being confined to a torture chamber for a second time. However, by moving a step at a time, each of them was released from their timeless convictions so that reality could impinge, and the shift took place. Later this had to be reworked when at 19 the only possible placement for further education and development acceptable to the parents involved Holly going to live in a community 40 miles away, where the expectation was that residents spent a good many weekends within the community. My capacity to defend the continuity of Holly's therapy over these changes seemed to help Mother believe that all would not be lost.

The final area of work I want to comment on took shape only in the last two years of Holly's therapy, and I believe it came about once we had begun to think together about when her treatment would end. Mother began to use the sessions to share with her husband for the first time some of her own terrible family history. He had always known of Mother's older institutionalized schizophrenic sister – she, indeed, was the maternal grandmother's model of Holly's future unless everyone protected her by entering her mad world. What he had never known was that Mother's step-father (her own father having died when she was very young) was a paranoid schizophrenic who had terrified both his wife and her two daughters with his violent unpredictable outbursts. Mother's childhood had thus been lived in the shadow of a psychotic sister and a psychotic father figure. As I learnt this, I was deeply impressed by the bravery with which this woman had fought and was fighting for access to an ordinary non-mad world. Something she had found in our work helped her in this lifelong struggle and also enabled her to reach a new level of trust in her husband's love and solidity.

It may be useful to add two small technical notes. I found that I needed to allow 75 minutes for the meetings with this couple. To give adequate attention both to issues concerning Holly and to the unfolding of their own personalities was not possible within the 50-minute frame. Even then, it was usually very difficult to end sessions, although Father became able to help me by remaining aware of the passing of time, and gradually Mother too gained a sense of the structure of the session and could gather herself together to be ready to leave. She was often almost overwhelmed by emotion during the session, yet dignified in her effort to regain some composure with which to depart. The second point is that Mother was free to telephone me in between our appointments. She was respectful of this in not making very frequent calls, but it was difficult to manage the length of conversations when she did ring. She did so when she was very worried about an impending external change and its impact on Holly, and also when she felt she must tell me about a change in Holly which she knew was significant but could not herself understand. Touchingly, she rang me the week after Holly's final session to tell me that Holly was sad, that they had talked about it and that Holly had said to her, 'I want to be in that room so that I can talk to Mrs Rustin'. Mother was both afraid that Holly would not manage without me and also moved by Holly's lucid search for support from her.

Third clinical example

Now I will go on to describe a second model for this supportive work with parents. I am indebted to Judith Loose for this clinical material.

Mr and Mrs B, parents of a young autistic girl, were seen together weekly in parallel with their daughter's treatment. For a long time their worker felt defeated by the repetitive ruminative anxious flow of talk from Mother which would lead to Father's eyes glazing over and his withdrawal from involvement.

Mrs B lost her mother when she was a few months old. She had a poor relationship with her step-mother and hated her half-sister who is severely mentally ill. Mr B came to England after traumatizing war service.

The therapist found herself unable to imagine how this couple could have had children, as they seemed so disconnected. In the early part of a session taking place after about one year of treatment, there had been a lively moment sparked off by Mother's tart observation that their therapist had not taken half-terms last year but was doing so this term. Father had spoken of the misdiagnosis of a serious illness of his father's, and his belief that it was best to steer clear of doctors who make mistakes but lack humility. Mother had criticized the school's failure to provide Beth with clean pants after an accident – she had been sent home in a nappy. 'If they have spare nappies, why not spare pants?' There was reference to a happy family outing, and talk of Beth's new capacity for discrimination about food. Then the session continued with the therapist enquiring of Mother about her memories of family meals.

Mum said sadly that her main meal was school lunch. She then either had tea with her child minder – because her father came home later – or, after her father re-married, with her step-mother and her younger sister who was at that time just a baby. This last part was said with some coldness. The therapist asked about snacks. What did she do when she was hungry? She seemed grateful to be asked and told an amusing story of not being allowed to eat sweets when wearing school uniform. Mr B looked interested as if he had never heard this story. Mum acknowledged how different it was today for Alice, their older daughter, who bought crisps whenever she felt like it.

When Mr B was asked if he remembered childhood meals, he said with a smile that they were big ones, especially breakfast, and the family was all together, often including a grandparent. He seemed momentarily happy and continued talking about high school and university when he had had jobs on farms to earn extra money. He said that then he had eaten with the farm families. He mentioned that city jobs were hard to come by and he could always find work 'defoliating' once he had a good reputation. The therapist asked if he could explain 'defoliating'.

He seemed to come alive. He described the process of corn hybrids and pollination rows in an almost passionate way. He spoke about walking up and down the countless rows with a kind of rhythm, pulling back the husk leaves of each individual corn. Mrs B actually turned in her chair so that she was facing him for the first time ever. The therapist felt that she did not need to hold onto the details as he had been able to capture his wife's attention. She was looking at him with surprising warmth.

Discussion

I think this material brings out very beautifully a process taking place between these parents which is being presided over by their therapist. Husband and wife are becoming interested in each other's separate existence – time spent apart in past or present is felt to be enriching their relationship. The primitive deprivation and neediness within mother is less oppressive. The session seems to be giving them pleasure.

The technique the therapist had adopted to counter the mindless flow of words which had engulfed earlier sessions has three elements, all rooted in meticulous observation. First, she is quick to pick up the negative transference. She shows herself to have strength to deal with this, and this modifies Mrs B's infantile despair about being attended to, a consequence of the early loss of her mother and her feeling of having been too much for her mother. There is some introjective identification with a competent adult in Mr and Mrs B's belated efforts to toilet-train Beth. Second, she interrupts Mrs B when repetitive stories appear, in an effort to hold Mr B's interest and to convey that Mrs B can be contained and that Mr B's active presence in the sessions is valued. Third, she expresses active interest in and curiosity about the thoughts and feelings of each of the parents. This gives the message of the importance of their different life stories and of the possibility of an enriched conversation when each person can be listened to. Once the therapist had allowed herself to become more actively curious, she was able to discover that Beth had been sleeping in her parents' room up to this point. Following some discussion of this, Mrs B reported a family weekend away when she had made up an extension bed next to theirs in the holiday hotel but noticed that Beth wanted to look at the twin bed next to Alice's. Mother had taken the point of this. This enquiring attitude of the therapist requires that care is taken to achieve a clear understanding – when she does not understand, she persists. This counters the tendency within families with an autistic member for experience of clear and rewarding communication to atrophy and for misunderstandings to abound. Mr B makes an implicit comparison between his experience of Mrs L, the therapist, who knows what she is doing and earlier experience of doctors which had been so unsatisfactory.

I think as child psychotherapists we are well suited to do the kind of work just described (Barrows, 1995). Our attunement to the infantile in our patients allows us access to the disturbance in adult and parental functioning which needs to be addressed. This case is an example of work where our own parental capacities – for taking responsibility for protecting vulnerability, for challenging self-destructive behaviour, for interesting ourselves in the everyday details of children's lives – are called upon. Such work may serve to give a first experience to deprived adults of attentive and thoughtful parental behaviour.

Work to promote change in family functioning

Now I shall move to discuss the cluster of cases where there is an agreed explicit aim of change within the family. This might lead to marital therapy or family therapy as such, but I would like to note one kind of work which I think appropriately attracts child psychotherapists. This is individual psychotherapeutic work with a parent, where there is a particular emphasis on clarifying the projections occurring between family members. This can be seen as analogous in some ways to psychoanalytically based family therapy (Copley, 1987). Such work makes use of transference in the therapeutic relationship, but the emphasis is more firmly focused on exploring the transferences within the family, with the aim of improving emotional containment. This can free the parent to function in a parental mode and the child to be less burdened with intergenerational difficulties.

Fourth clinical example

I shall now present a clinical illustration. My work with Miss D, a single mother who had adopted John at age six, began when John was 14. Mother and son had been seen together from time to time by the child psychiatrist who had been involved in the original adoption placement. In early adolescence, John became very angry and upset. He was doing badly at school, increasingly involved with delinquent gang-life and drug culture, and out of control at home. He was extremely abusive to mother and stole from her on a large scale.

My psychiatrist colleague asked me to see mother while she continued with John, following an episode when he smashed a picture in an explosion of rage during a joint session. The initial nine months were a time of real turbulence. John was admitted to an adolescent in-patient unit for a while, and mother was desperate and frightened much of the time. She gradually became able to reassert her authority, gained support when needed from the local police, and came to understand that she could not allow John to live at home if he persisted in theft from and violence towards her. Eventually he was housed in an excellent hostel with a key-worker support system.

I shall present some recent material which is characteristic of the mix of themes tackled in this once-weekly work. Miss D is an unusual person. She is an intelligent and imaginative woman with many gifts, but there have been great impediments in her making use of these in her life. Her history is important in understanding this. She is the child of German Jewish refugees who escaped from Berlin in 1938. Many of their relatives died in the Holocaust. She had one brother who died in his early 30s. She has not married, although she has had some very close relationships with men, and has many friends.

After some months of crisis-driven work, it became clear to me that she needed psychotherapy in her own right. I talked to her about this, making it clear that this would be a different experience from what had happened so far. I added that she might prefer me to refer her to a separate service, since the Child and Family Department perhaps felt like a place for her and John together. However, if she wished, I would be able to work with her on this changed basis, since we had already come to understand a good deal together and might build on this. We agreed to end our weekly meetings, leaving her two months in which she could think things over. My vacancy would be available from the following term if she decided to take it up.

She accepted my offer, though giving me a taste of what was to come by falling violently in love on a trip abroad, which entailed cancelling our first two sessions of the term.

John is now 18. Miss D had an accident last December in which she broke her leg badly. She had to miss the last session before Christmas, and most of January, because she was immobilized. She then returned on two crutches. It was clear to both of us that this accident was linked to beginning to think about the end of therapy – the fall was a consequence of her missing the last step on the stairs and seemed to represent her anxiety that facing the end was a time of danger for her, of not feeling safely held inside.

In the session I want to refer to, she began by noticing that, in the sink in my room, John's name is engraved in metal (the sink-maker's trademark). She smiled and said he might not like that. She went on to describe her journey to my room and her thought as she struggled along the corridor – I don't want to be a patient any more, not at the

Tavistock or the Whittington (a local hospital). She felt she would never get to the first floor and could not bear her dependence on the lift, on the receptionist to tell me she was here, on the woman who did not help her by holding the swing doors or on me who decided when she could come. She was feeling very wobbly, she added.

I linked this to our recognition that the end of her therapy was now going to be talked about between us, leaving her in a rush to get away, and yet wobbly and needy. She went on to talk about John, who is serving a six-week prison sentence. She had been very worried about him this week, knowing that his phone calls were leaving something out. Eventually he told her that he had been in a fight and had been locked up in solitary confinement for a week. She movingly described the circumstances – he had been reading ('You'll never believe this, Mum', he told her) and had been taunted by a group of young men, and this ended up in fighting. He said it had been awful, but he had coped. He had a long talk with the governor, who said that he was not the sort of young man who should be in prison. She spoke of his negotiating to have some unpaid fines dealt with as part of his prison sentence, so that he could start with a clean slate when he came out. 'John is so balanced, in the way he is trying to work this out', she said, and grinned as she thought of her own huge efforts to keep her balance.

> I offered to help him with the fines and said I did not want him to be in prison longer, but he wrote to me that he wanted to sort it out himself and that it would be all right. But somehow he thinks I have the key.

I spoke about her confusion – she wishes to be in my mind, engraved there like John's name on my sink, but then gets frightened that I will not let her go, might imprison her. She finds it so difficult to believe, when she feels me to be a mother who needs to hold on to her, that she can also find a father-aspect of me who might help her to feel ready to leave. I talked at some length about the idea of being held in my mind as a living separate being who would end her therapy here and go on to live her life as I would my own.

She went on to talk about her fatherless nephew for whom she often provides counsel, and the theme of finding father's voice was explored in relation to John, to her nephew and in the transference, and she then talked about her own father's role in supporting her during her university years. 'But later on he couldn't help me', she mused. To her own amazement she found herself recalling sitting at a café frequented by German refugees where she would meet her father when she came to live and work in London. He brought a book to show her, Victor Zorza's account of his daughter's death from cancer. She spoke movingly of her parents' complete inability to talk to each other about their son's illness and death, and her father describing to her the comfort of reading this book and asking her to read it too, but never to speak to her mother about it.

Later she connected this unshared and incomplete mourning with the recent funeral of an aunt, and her nephew's wish to visit his father's grave, and for the headstone to be altered to include him.

I described her longing to bring together the strong father aspect of me with whom she felt these tragedies, like those of the refugees in the café, could be shared and the mother aspect, to confront the idea that she always had to take a protective role towards me and not speak of her wish to end therapy and leave me. I linked this to her pre-Christmas accident, and showed her that she feels it is very dangerous to herself to live in accordance with this belief. I described her hope that she could encounter in me a sense of mother and father in communication with each other.

The session ended with her speaking of how, after her aunt's death, she had talked for the first time to her mother about all the family members who died in the camps. She found out that her mother did know their names, where they had been killed and buried. A friend going to Auschwitz recently had sought out their names and said Kaddish for them.

She said, 'I came back here to find a different way to leave', and I agreed that this was so. I had myself been feeling during her January absence that helping her to get back so that an ending could take place was going to be a difficult task.

This material is much condensed, but I think it does illustrate what I mean about the multi-layered work that we can sometimes do in working with parents. Despite John's continuing difficulties, the two of them have re-established a real relationship. When he heard of her accident, he came rushing to the hospital at once, and in a recent letter from prison he said he had realized that she was not only a good mum, but also a good friend to him. Her part in this great change has been to struggle with huge personal difficulties in establishing a separate identity, to give up a predominantly manic defensive system, and to sort out the unmourned dead, who haunted her dreams, from the child adopted in part because he represented the necessity to rescue the abandoned Jews who had not escaped. Inevitably, the details of her family story revealed a terrible toll of guilt. This work has left a space in which she and her son have begun to get to know each other in a fresh way.

Referral outside the child and family setting

Sometimes we find ourselves referring a parent with major difficulties to an adult psychotherapist or analyst outside the child and family psychiatric setting. One of the disadvantages of this is that there may be rather little attention to the damaging projective processes going on in the family in the present. Within the Tavistock, we have found that referrals to the Adult Department for psychotherapy of a parent sometimes create a painful split between the priority given to the infantile needs of the patient and the protection required for vulnerable children and young people. When an adult patient is being seen within an adult psychotherapy service, the attention paid to the impact of the patient's internal difficulties on parental functioning is less to the fore. Psychotherapy provided within the child and family setting, and by therapists with experience of work with children, tends to be particularly attuned to the interferences in adult relational capacities which are consequent on infantile anxieties and phantasies, and to concentrate on delineating and differentiating adult from infantile aspects of the personality (Harris, 1968). This approach, which depends on a firm gathering of the infantile transference within the therapy, is supportive of improved parental functioning.

Ethical issues

Finally I should like to share a few reflections on ethical issues raised in work with parents. There are two areas of concern: one is when there is a refusal on the part of parents to take their children's welfare seriously; the second is where therapy with the parent may endanger their capacity to sustain adult functioning.

When we are faced with clear cases of abuse of children, we can usually resolve how to proceed, although the limited resources of social services and the clumsiness of the law can be a troubling disincentive. More tricky are examples of emotional abuse. A case in point would be the following: I found myself working with a couple, well-known in the local community as public figures, in relation to the therapy of their adopted son Robert. Robert was failing at school and stole things at home. He denied these acts of theft resolutely. In his therapy, there was soon a defensive impasse. In my work with the couple I learnt that the magistrate father was blackmailing mother not to speak about problems in the family relationships – his sanction was to absent himself from our meetings and thereafter to withdraw support for the child's therapy. On one occasion they brought a small model made by Robert who was very good at art. It was a highly disturbing devil figure, clearly related to father's looks. Father demonstrated his pride in his son's technical capacity, and his lack of awareness of the reference to himself, and then proceeded to use the model as evidence that his son would go to the bad. He took the devil image as concrete evidence of the 'bad blood' which the child had inherited from his aberrant natural parents. The cold rejection and lack of concern for the boy's future in his attitude was breathtaking. In due course, I learnt from Mother, who returned in a more desperate state sometime after the ending of Robert's unsatisfactory therapy, that the family was based on a profound lie – Father was carrying on a secret affair with a woman on the staff of the court, and denying the truth of this when she confronted him. He was in fact as determined a liar as Robert.

The work it was possible to do was very limited. Mother was too frightened of the loss of her social position and relative economic security to force the issue with her husband. Meanwhile, the corrosive effects of this hypocritical situation on the children were serious. Robert's delinquent behaviour had escalated, Father's attitude combined cynical despair with vicarious enjoyment of Robert's dangerous lifestyle. I tried to help Mother to take seriously the price being paid for the maintenance of this dishonest structure, and she pulled herself out of some of her self-destructive collusive behaviour.

Fifth clinical example

A different kind of ethical issue arises when we are faced with a parent at risk of breakdown. A recent case illustrates this well. I am grateful to Biddy Youell for this material. Mrs C is an experienced foster mother. She was being seen once a week at the clinic to support her in the care of two very seriously abused children and to sustain her commitment to bringing them to therapy. The children are aged eight and six.

The crisis I want to describe occurred following Mrs C's decision to adopt the children. She took them to visit her mother and brother in New Zealand over Christmas, and returned saying she could no longer cope with their difficult behaviour and wanted them removed. Social Services were horrified, as Mrs C had been seen as a tower of strength who could cope with anything. They offered extra support, but also told Mrs C that, if she could not cope, then the children would have to go into institutional care. This made her feel very guilty. The Social Services Department was in a panic because these children had been abused both sexually and physically while in care in two previous foster homes. This had led to court cases, and several social workers had been disciplined for negligence.

Mrs C's therapist found herself struggling with very painful conflicting questions. The children's therapist as well as Social Services wanted Mrs C to be persuaded to hold on to them, but Mrs C's therapist had before her a woman in a state of extreme emotional collapse, beneath the façade of rejection and blame of the children. Their behaviour had regressed while they were on holiday, and her relatives had been disgusted by them. Quite soon Mrs C acknowledged that she knew she was ill. She shivered, hunched in silent tears, and spoke of how she felt unable to take the antidepressants prescribed by her GP for fear that the pills would take away her last vestiges of control. She feared falling into the state of mind of the time when she was widowed. She described nightmares of hundreds of worms and of driving into a black hole.

The therapist was aware that Mrs C had been a coper all her life. She had found a solution to her own early deprivation in becoming a super-competent carer. This identity had collapsed and it was evident that she could not care for the children at this point. The painful question was how to maintain proper concern for her mental health. She needed some protection from the demands of child care professionals who could not bear her breakdown. Additionally, the therapist felt anxious that her weekly supportive work with Mrs C might have contributed to her becoming more open to her fragile underlying emotional state and have undermined her very rigid defences.

This case therefore raised the issue of our judgement about when defences need to be supported – for example might it have been wiser to accept Mrs C's initial assertion that once a month sessions would be fine for her? When we work with parents who are themselves very deprived or have other borderline features, keeping the temperature of the involvement cool may sometimes be wise. The support systems we build for our work with adults are one of the crucial elements in giving us a sense of proper professional authority.

Conclusion

People who want to train and work as child psychotherapists usually have a profound identification with the child's point of view. This perspective provides us with ready access to the child aspects of our adult patients' personalities. When there is an opportunity to do psychotherapeutic work using the infantile transference we have rich experience to draw on. This has to be married with an awareness of other issues in adult lives, and in adult psychotherapy. Nonetheless, the intensive training in psychoanalytic work with children and young people provides a very strong base from which to tackle this work. The passionate conflicts of family life are what bring parents to seek our help, and often the pain opened up by troubles between parents and children provides an appropriate opening for facing fundamental issues. We sometimes have an exceptional opportunity to help and need to have the confidence to do so.

13

WORK WITH PARENTS (1999/2021)

Introduction

The context for thinking about the range of work done by child psychotherapists with parents has changed greatly since my earlier paper about this and since the first edition of the *Handbook of Child and Adolescent Psychotherapy* was published in 1999. This is particularly the case with respect to work done within NHS Child and Adolescent Mental Health Services and other publicly funded settings providing family support. The full implications of the many changes in public policy and the changing shape of services continue to be worked out, but it is striking that public and governmental preoccupation with parenting is at a consistently high level. For example, commissioners of child and adolescent mental health services are expected to develop a 'parenting strategy' and to plan services accordingly. If we turn to the evidence provided by column inches in the press and the numbers of television programmes about parenting, we are confronted by ongoing anxious preoccupation, a significant tendency to blame parents, and an emphasis on the need to educate and support parents in their responsibilities. The challenge for child psychotherapists is to locate their practice within this active discourse on parenting. What is the particular contribution that we can make? What opportunities are there to influence thinking more broadly? What new services are likely to develop in the current conjuncture? What about the evidence base for traditional child psychotherapy approaches to work with parents? Most importantly, what are the growing points of clinical practice and the questions our psychoanalytic framework of understanding can enable us to explore?

DOI: 10.4324/9781003325543-18

It is worth bearing in mind that a significant proportion of child psychotherapists undertake further training either as family, couple or individual adult psychotherapists. Perhaps one reason for this trend is the interest in work with parents and the conviction of its importance. Within the core initial training, there is a relatively small though significant requirement for such experience. In the clinical context, however, there is a continuing problem in finding colleagues from other disciplines able to provide long-term input for parents. This is partly due to a lack within CAMHS teams of experience of working in a way which attends to unconscious factors and makes use of transference phenomena as they emerge in the clinical setting. The public sector emphasis on brief interventions as the preferred service framework makes it hard to justify more extensive support for parents. The IMPACT research study did however provide an opportunity for some new forms of inter-disciplinary thinking about parent work (Cregeen *et al.*, 2017). However, while short-term interventions have the laudable aim of ensuring that professional resources reach a much wider population and that waiting lists are reduced, they have a problematic impact on the provision of and effectiveness of child psychotherapy. One thing the evidence base (Kennedy, 2003; Trowell *et al.*, 2007) makes clear is that parallel work with parents is as important as we have always believed. This means that skilled practitioners are needed to undertake such work if child psychotherapy is to achieve its aims. In some settings, family therapists, social workers, psychologists and other colleagues are able to provide this, but it seems increasingly the case that this cannot be relied on, and that child psychotherapists now need to take on the role of parent worker more frequently. This can be a very potent and enjoyable co-operative effort, but it raises two obvious questions for the profession. The first is the issue of confidence and competence in parent work, and the second is that of the balance of different forms of clinical work – work with children and adolescents, work with parents, family work, short and long term work. If the demand for work with parents is growing, it has implications for the primary identity of child psychotherapists and for training.

The twenty-first century parent is living in a world very different indeed from that of fifty years ago and the early days of child psychotherapy. The majority of mothers are at work through much of their children's childhood, the number of single parents has increased enormously, and divorce and family break up is much more common. Looking beyond the immediate family context, things are also much changed – the support of extended families is less available, due in part to geographical mobility; competitive and stressful aspects of the education system are writ large; and the impact of the visual and consumerist culture of television, the internet and social media is enormous. The multi-cultural and multi-ethnic neighbourhoods of our cities, the fearfulness with respect to children's safety in public spaces, the earlier incidence of puberty and changes in patterns of reproduction, including all the possibilities for assisted pregnancy, are other significant factors. The rate of social and technological change is awe inspiring, yet the human capacity for responding to change is a well-recognized area of psychological vulnerability. It is therefore by no means surprising that this is a period in which people struggle to make sense of what is happening. There may indeed be a degree of mis-attunement between the rate of technological change and the pace at which human beings can adapt their forms of life to the new conditions. The extent of uncertainty about what parents should be doing and the now widespread idea that they need to be taught how to be parents suggests both the destabilizing effect of so much change on traditional identities, on a socially accepted notion of what it is to be a parent, and the fact that our society approaches its human problems in a technical spirit. Confused or failing parents are thought to require cognitive psychological techniques to fill the gap. The popularity of 'Super-Nanny' approaches is an aspect of this, as is the widespread enthusiasm for parenting classes.

This background is very important in understanding what parents are troubled by; what they expect, hope or fear from professionals; and similarly vital in thinking about what commissioners of services are looking for and what partnerships between health, social care and education services and voluntary agencies might work. Although this book is written with clinical practice at its heart, attention to the wider context seems to me to be essential if our clinical work is to be responsive to the inner world implications for our patients of ongoing social change. We need to be in good ongoing dialogue with colleagues, researchers and the wider public in debating what is helpful for parents in difficulties with each other and their children.

'Parenting strategy' is a phrase one comes across in many policy documents, including for example the report on the implementation of the National Service Framework with respect to children's mental health (Shribman, 2007). The interpretation given to the 'Every Child Matters' agenda was that all the agencies involved were to devise such a strategy, and one of the particular points made was the welcome emphasis on the needs of children whose parents have mental illness. Although such joined-up thinking lost its influence as governments changed, the more recent heightened concern about young people's mental health may create fresh opportunities. Nonetheless, the predominant tone remains one to do with information and education for parents, through the provision of 'parent-management programmes' and training, for foster and kinship carers, for example. Advice lines for parents seem to be quite well used, and social media parental self-help initiatives have proved popular. Overall the emphasis tends to be on providing information, but the listening skills of telephone counsellors and the sharing of experiences between parents offer something of greater emotional depth.

Partnership is another concept espoused very broadly, and this is a tricky idea in the clinical context. At one level, one can be sure that unless a partnership is achieved between clinician and a child's parents, there is no basis for useful work – there has to be some trust, some agreement about what is wrong and what might be done about it. The old language of consent and therapeutic alliance is another way of describing this process. But as used currently, partnership can come to mean something rather different. The idea of parents choosing from a menu of what is available places the whole interchange at a consumerist and narrowly cognitive level and leaves to one side the meaning of the relationship that is being established as soon as a conversation about family difficulties is started. The unconscious is being ruled out as a significant factor once partnership is interpreted in a way which is designed to avoid recognizing dependence on the therapist, and to assert equality, when the reality is that one person needs something that the other may be able to help them find. The 'partnership' discourse is related to the issue of rights, and the right of patients to be fully informed and to be given choices is sometimes interpreted in such a way as to reduce their right to be understood, looked after and given what is appropriate from the point of view of professional expertise. Interestingly, this confusion is quite similar to the problem of thinking about children's rights – parents can become so taken over by ideas of a child's right to have whatever they wish that they lose a sense of the authority and responsibility they have as adults to consider whether what the child would choose is good for him or not.

The concept of anxiety is what seems to be missing from much of the parenting discourse, and it is one without which the experience of parents cannot be properly described. This is odd, since what parents so often feel are anxieties of many kinds, sometimes fairly ordinary and sometimes quite overwhelming. Whether we are thinking of the parents of a distressed or ill baby, a defiant toddler, a bullied school-child, a depressed or acting-out or anorexic adolescent, what all are struggling with is their worry, panic or despair. There is a continuity between the absolutely unavoidable everyday anxieties of being a parent and the extreme ones, which bring families to the attention of child psychotherapists. It is when the level of anxiety bursts through the parents' capacity to contain it that outside help is sought, but it is very helpful to keep in mind that it is ordinary and necessary for parents to be worried about their children. If we put it in the language of attachment, we might suggest that normal secure attachment is indeed the child's link to someone who is capable of being anxious about the child. Bion's understanding of the vital role of maternal reverie in the development of the capacity for thought gives a deeper account of the role which primary dependence plays in the development of a person. It is a mind which can register the child's anxiety which is the starting point of everything, and parents in trouble are very often in difficulties with respect to this function.

There are some other central psychoanalytic concepts which underpin child psychotherapists' styles of work with parents which can be usefully outlined at this point. Some of these concepts would be shared by therapists working within different conceptual frameworks, though perhaps differently understood when the unconscious dimension of mental life is taken into account.

The distinction between infantile and adult states of mind is a bedrock for thinking developmentally. It is all too easy to observe times when parental functioning, which requires adult capacities, is undermined because of overwhelming infantile feelings and phantasies. Finding a way to help parents to become aware of this process in themselves and thus be able to protect themselves is probably our most cherished aim. A second dimension is our characterization of maternal and paternal aspects of personality and parental functioning. Very broadly this describes two necessary forms of parental behaviour – the receptive, nurturing and more relationally oriented maternal mode and the limit-setting, paternal mode with its greater focus on the outside world, the child's ambitions and curiosity and potential achievements. The balance of these within individuals and the way in which they are distributed in a parental couple is a fruitful vertex of development. The third vital set of ideas is the Oedipus complex and its sequelae. The sexual tie between parents is an aspect of their relationship which is often difficult for their children but also difficult for professionals to pay attention to when their prime focus of attention is on the parent/child relationship. The couple element of the parental couple can sometimes be the key to the family difficulties, a point perhaps more often recognized when the couple relationship has broken down and the task of the separated pair is to find a way of continuing to function as parents. This may be rendered painfully problematic when feelings of sexual rejection and jealousy intrude, as they often do, when new partners enter the picture. The increasing numbers of reconstituted families with step-parents, step and half siblings add an additional complexity. Finally, the experience of shame among parents who need help with their children is a significant clinical problem – their sense of failure and incompetence, and their dread of feeling despised and humiliated by those seen as more successful at being grown-up is a severe hindrance in parent work. Linked to this is unconscious envy, with its corrosive impact on relationships which stir up a sense of need.

The complexities of confidentiality in clinical work should be mentioned here as it impacts on relationships with parents as patients in very difficult ways. When there is already some involvement with the law or statutory bodies at the outset, taking the legal context – child protection issues, domestic violence, family court proceedings etc – into account is built in. When, however, the origin of the referral lies elsewhere and the family expects full confidentiality, there can be great strain and anxiety on both sides if issues erupt or revelations get made which require a statutory response. The current expectation for more and more inter-agency co-work and for rather routine sharing of much information throws up increasingly difficult decisions for professionals and raises tricky challenges to accepted practice.

Here is part of the overview of child psychotherapists' approaches to work with parents I wrote for the first edition of the handbook, together with some reflective comments. It was not a blueprint for a parenting service but rather a depiction of some kinds of work with parents which child psychotherapists are equipped to do.

Consultation with parents

The traditional role for the child psychotherapist limited contact with parents to meetings, held from time to time, to review a child's progress in therapy. Their purpose was to sustain a co-operative relationship between therapist and parents, to give the therapist a sense of the child's development in the family, at school and in the wider social world, and the parents an opportunity to enquire about the therapy and test out their confidence in the therapist's capacity to help their child. At their best, such meetings can offer a real chance to integrate diverse perspectives and to enrich the understanding of both parents and therapist, but they can also be difficult occasions in which divergences in aim between therapist and parent may erupt. Such reviews remain an important part of good practice.

Two examples will serve to illustrate these points.

Case example: Jacob

Jacob is a ten-year-old boy referred by divorced parents who remain very angry with each other, but who have managed to co-operate in supporting Jacob's therapy. He was referred for extremely aggressive and disruptive behaviour at school, which was threatening to lead to his exclusion, and for his difficult and unrewarding family relationships. His rigid defences made him rather inaccessible to help and his therapist found it hard to sustain hope in the face of a barrage of contempt from Jacob. Termly review meetings were held with each parent separately as neither felt able to sustain parental concern in company with the other. When the issue of choice of secondary school arose, parental conflict flared up, and there was potential for Jacob's much improved behaviour at school (his problems now being gathered, and more or less contained, in his relationship with his therapist) to be undermined. The review meetings could be used to support the more adult aspect of the parents' personalities and thus enable them to think about Jacob's needs at school rather than be drawn into another fight at his expense. The therapist's observations about Jacob's vulnerability to being upset by changes, his need for careful preparation and explanation, and his well-concealed panic about what secondary school would be like, helped them to hold back and work out their differences less flagrantly.

Comment

Trying to place work of this sort in the context of service development, one might want to draw attention to the importance of sustaining the involvement of father in families where parents have separated. In this particular family, Jacob's difficulties in managing his aggressive feelings and in differentiating between ordinary self-assertion, bullying, and risky or delinquent challenges to adult authority meant that his need for paternal attention, especially during the adolescent years, was likely to be intense.

It is interesting to note that developments in psychoanalytic theorizing about fathers, male and female elements in the personality, and maternal and paternal aspects of parental functioning have been growing over a number of years (Trowell & Etchegoyen, 2002; Britton, 1998; Houzel, 2001; Morgan, 2019) and the interest in parents as couples is now a significant area of couple psychotherapy. This may enable child psychotherapists to work more confidently with parental couples in conflict, and indeed more are undertaking specific training as couple therapists (Cregeen, 2017).

Case example: Elizabeth

Elizabeth is an adopted girl, aged nine, with a very sad and disrupted early life. She attends for intensive psychotherapy. Review meetings frequently provided rather crucial opportunities to test out realities. Elizabeth would often give a very convincing account to her therapist of external events which would interfere with her clinic appointments, leaving the therapist in doubt as to what was going to happen. Her parents, similarly, would hear disturbing stories about school and therapy whose reality they could not assess. Exploration suggested that Elizabeth was not telling lies in any ordinary sense, but rather conveying both how hard it was for her to distinguish between reality and fantasy and how doubtful she was that adults could co-operate and stick to arrangements made for her benefit. In her first five years, she had little experience of consistent adult care and she continued to recreate opportunities to be let down, when her conviction that people did not really care would be confirmed.

Helping Elizabeth's parents not to be pulled into rejecting behaviour was facilitated by the exploration of the details of her difficult behaviour. For example, Father complained of her tendency to scream right into his ear, but was helped to think about this symptom when we could identify the painful intensity and shock which she was forcing him to experience on her behalf. Perhaps this might be likened to the ordinary behaviour of a crying infant, but when the baby gets no response the screams stay lodged in the baby's head in an unbearable way. Seeing the baby within the nine-year-old helped Elizabeth's parents to find ways to cope with her.

Comment

Work with adopted and fostered children has become an increasingly large part of child psychotherapy practice as has been widely acknowledged. The question of how to respond to the difficulties their parents face has led to many creative initiatives. (Cregeen, 2017). Elizabeth's parents were seen regularly as a parental couple, in addition to the review meetings discussed, by a co-worker of the child's therapist. But the complex problems of parenting children who have usually had a traumatic start in life and whose capacity for basic trust is deeply compromised often require new forms of help. These can include groups of parents in similar circumstances, often combining some information giving and behavioural strategy emphasis with ongoing support; a telephone conversation service for emergency use (particularly relevant for foster carers whose lives are so frequently disrupted by emergency placements); and careful long-term work with adoptive parents or family therapy prior to any consideration of individual treatment for their troubled children. Adoptive parents are very vulnerable to feeling that their own capacities are being undervalued or that they are being blamed for difficulties the children brought with them from their earlier lives. Hence, sensitivity to these anxieties is needed and timing of interventions is a delicate matter.

Individual work

The supportive work with parents, very often provided in the past by psychiatric social workers, is now more frequently undertaken by child psychotherapists themselves. This may be alongside a child's therapy taken on by another therapist, or as an intervention in its own right, because the most helpful input is deemed to be work aimed at changing parental functioning. A considerable variety of approach is required in this work. The spectrum includes support for quite disturbed parents whose own mental state may impinge in damaging ways on their children, support for deprived and vulnerable parents (for example, bereaved families, mothers abandoned by their partners, refugee families), and work which attempts to explore ways in which parental functioning is disturbed by unconscious aspects of the parents' own way of seeing things (Bailey, 2006). The balance of listening and receptiveness on the one hand, and insight-giving interventions on the other will depend on what a particular parent seems likely to be most helped by. Some fragile parents may be able to take in very little reflective comment and have urgent need for a relationship within which they can express their confusion, depression, despair and self-doubt, and feel that they can be accepted as they are. Others, with some source of greater hopefulness within their personality, will respond to the opportunity to think in-depth about their own contribution to their children's problems, and to consider their own family history as part of an attempt to understand the current family difficulties.

In working with parents, the therapist offers a model of how to respond to emotional distress which has some core elements. The first is attention to establishing and maintaining a reliable setting in which it is possible to talk about very upsetting things. As with a child's treatment, sessions for parents have regularity in time and space, and this helps to contain the infantile elements which are aroused. The second element is the co-creation of some shared language to describe painful emotional states. Finding words for anguish is a help in itself, because it provides the comfort of feeling understood and therefore not alone with one's pain. Many lonely or emotionally deprived parents discover resources for understanding their own children through the experience of feeling understood and acquiring ways of thinking about feelings which may be very new to them. Third is the valuing of boundaries and differentiation: the differences between parents and children, and between adult and more infantile aspects of the personality, can be clarified within a structured therapeutic setting. For example, an emotionally deprived parent can find it very difficult to distinguish between need and greed in herself and her child: if primary needs have never been met

220

adequately, setting limits which are not arbitrary is almost impossible. Fourth is an adequately complex understanding of human emotion and intimate relationships. This involves exploration of the internal world and of the constraints and creative possibilities of external reality. To support the development of genuine parental functioning, attention has to be given not only to the individual but also to the marital relationship – where there is a partnership – to the role of work in the individual's identity, to the full range of family relationships across the generations and to the community setting. Last, and most important, there is the focus on giving meaning to behaviour. The urge to blame and reject aspects of ourselves and others is most helpfully modified if our destructive impulses can be given meaning.

Case example: Mrs C

Mrs C was a divorced woman in her early fifties with two sons. The older, aged 26, was on the edge of a third schizophrenic breakdown when Mrs C referred herself and her younger boy, Tobias, aged 14, for help. It quickly became clear that the help Tobias wanted was that someone should take care of his troubled mother and relieve him of a very heavy burden of anxiety. Mrs C began once-weekly psychotherapy. Her concerns for her two sons were deeply interwoven with the overall pattern of her life. She had had two significant sexual relationships and each had produced a child, but neither father had a reliable relationship to his son or with her. Mrs C's struggle to find an identity of her own and emerge from compliance with what she felt had been an authoritarian and rather loveless family had contributed to her choice of partner, as each of them had represented a counter-cultural protest against the restrictions she so resented. Now she was struggling with two enormous anxieties: her schizophrenic son exploited her ruthlessly, stealing from her and taking a very unfair share of the emotional and physical space she tried to provide. How could she stand up to him? As she became more in touch with the anger she had never expressed to her own parents, whose work abroad had resulted in her being sent to a boarding school from age five, she developed a capacity to challenge him. Her second concern was her own health. She had had two life-threatening illnesses in the last five years and was anxious that her younger son might have to cope with her early death.

Thinking about this meant facing all her own painful losses. The depression this precipitated took her deep into herself. Gradually Mrs C became more able to acknowledge and value her feelings, including those that made her feel guilty, and less prone to see them in others. Her creative capacities began to re-emerge.

Comment

A major current public health concern is the impact of parental mental illness on the development of children. This case highlights the reverse issue of how families cope with mental illness in children and young people. The individual work offered to Mrs C was once characterized by a child psychiatry colleague as 'family therapy done via individual psychotherapy', which makes a cogent point. The child psychotherapist's perspective is an inclusive one, because it acknowledges family dynamics – everyone in the family system is affected by everyone else. The choice of whom to help is usually a mixture of pragmatics (who is asking for it? – Mrs C was, her son was not, being understandably anxious not to seem psychologically ill, like his brother) and resources. The provision of psychotherapy for parents as an integral part of Child and Adolescent services seems to me a priority which is currently almost totally neglected. Referral to adult services tends to lead to loss of the capacity to bear the child in mind and less attention to ongoing parental projections into the children.

Case example: Mr J

Mr J was a father of two boys, the older of whom was autistic. He was troubled by his own deep passivity in the face of his son's regressed behaviour. He and his wife were initially seen jointly to talk about their children's difficulties: the younger son's omnipotent and manic behaviour seemed to complement his brother's autistic withdrawal from life, and the parents became aware that the division of labour between the boys and between the two of them was at the expense of all of them as individuals. Mr and Mrs J were offered individual help to understand this destructive process. As Mr J talked, he began to see that his two sons were confused in his mind with himself and his younger brother. This brother had had a heart condition from birth, and Mr J had given up much of his ordinary childhood desires to take care of him. This had evoked hatred of which he had been unaware, and when his brother died he had been left with a burden of guilt which lay heavily on his early adult years. His own child's autism and consequent need for special care had been experienced as just punishment. The younger son was left to express the ambition and longing for life and the anger which Mr J had had to disown.

Comment

Psychotherapeutic services for autistic children and their families are often very deeply appreciated by the small number who receive them, as many publications have demonstrated (Alvarez, 1992; Klauber, 1998; Alvarez & Reid, 1999; Rhode, 2008). Concern about the poor quality of mental health provision for children with a learning disability has led to some real development, but there may be a tendency for relative neglect of parental need, especially if the children are offered therapy in school contexts. Mr J's preoccupation with intergenerational pressures may be especially relevant given the genetic element in childhood autism.

The possibility of preventative early intervention in this area is suggested by the pilot research in using a form of infant observation to support the mother–toddler relationship when autistic phenomena are emerging (Gretton, 2006). The potential for the therapeutic use of observation in the home is one which combines provision for parent and child.

I now want to add a category of work I did not discuss in my original paper. The significant expansion of interest in couple therapies suggests what a major omission this was.

The couple as focus

A focus which can sometimes seem the obvious one, despite the referral being of a child, is that of difficulties in the couple relationship. This can be quite a challenge for child psychotherapists unless they have had additional training, but a psychoanalytic understanding of couple problems can be so fruitful that it is an area of work ripe for development, especially in the context of greater contemporary openness in acknowledging relationship difficulties. Relationship counselling often does not include much attention to the place of the children in the family dynamics, but the destructive impact of couple conflict, domestic violence and other less obvious signs of breakdown in family relationships is enormous.

Working with the couple is bound to involve marital and sexual aspects alongside the problematic identity as parents. Here is one example of couple work which includes the therapist's concerns about the child.

Case example: Mr and Mrs A

This couple were 'semi-separated', the husband having moved next door to what had been intended as the family home when it was bought ten years ago. A large derelict Georgian house, bought with the aim of renovation had remained untouched while they lived next door in a tiny flat. The wife complained that her husband never really consulted her about the plans and he felt she dreamt up impractical schemes which could never be carried out. As a result of this impasse, their belongings had never been unpacked and their flat remained jam packed with crates and boxes. There was no room to move, literally or metaphorically. They were in a stalemate. They were neither living in or out of the marriage.

Mrs A poured out grievances and Mr A defended himself with terse replies. He was very silent, ponderous and seemingly impenetrable, while Mrs A would either scream with complaints about his inactivity or remain silent, tight lipped and out of reach. They both complained that they were not listened to, but were completely unaware of their own deafness to each other. They have an eight-year-old daughter who moves between them. The daughter was a go-between in many senses; she seemed to try to link them up. They competed for her attention, and both wanted to claim her as their own.

The more lively engaging aspects of themselves did however find expression in the relationship that they each had with their daughter. They both lightened up as they described her as 'a live wire', and she was a source of great pride. Her liveliness, they insisted, was an indication that she was fine. I realized my intense efforts to draw them out mirrored this. The couple told me that their daughter said that when she grew up she wanted to be a gardener; her dream was to have a garden of her own so she could nurture plants and flowers. Because of my own experience of desperately trying to inject some life into this couple I suddenly could identify with the enormous burden for her parents' growth that this little girl was carrying. She had been triangulated into her parents' relationship to link them up and bring some life and growth into a family scene that was so arid.

If this couple could be helped to gain some understanding of the nature of their relationship, there was a possibility that their daughter might be released from the burden she was carrying and become once more an eight-year-old girl whose parents could attend to her and not the other way round.

Group work

Some parents are more responsive to group therapy. The group offers the comfort that others, too, share a sense of failure, whether it be losing one's temper, failing to get a child to school on time or to bed at a reasonable hour, or trying to bear a child's failure at school, quarrelsomeness with siblings or antisocial behaviour. Group work seems to be helpful when there is a sense of social isolation, strong feelings of failure and an absence of supportive partners. The group culture, as long as the group does not contain deeply disturbed and destructive individuals, can create a place for each person's vulnerability and a sense of continuity over time as each member feels kept in mind by others. By and large, group work with parents builds on the constructive potential mobilized by the parental role and does not address so successfully negative factors, which are better tackled in the more protected space provided by individual work. This is because the members' identity as parents cannot be set on one side, as it might be in individual psychotherapy where their more infantile aspects can be contained. Parents do, however, challenge each other's evasions of responsibility, often with the help of humour.

Conclusion

Child psychotherapists in my view bring some special capacities to work with parents. The place of infant observation and the broad study of child development in their training, together with their own analysis, put them in touch with the changing pressures on parents as their children grow and develop, and the intensity with which parents' own infantile difficulties are stirred up by their children's emotional lives. This knowledge and sensitivity can be used well in responding to parental anxieties, but it can also be a source of trouble. A degree of competition, jealousy and envy is likely to be evoked by professionals who try to help when parents feel themselves to have failed. Tact, humility and a real belief in the shared nature of the task are essential. The direct use of transference and countertransference and interpretation are only appropriate when there has been explicit agreement that the parents wish to become patients in their own right. However, the understanding available through observation of the relationship made with the therapist can inform other kinds of conversation which have therapeutic potential. It is the capacity to empathize with both parental and child perspectives which is so valuable.

14

IDENTITY FRAGMENTATION AND RECOVERY IN PSYCHOANALYTIC PSYCHOTHERAPY (1989/2020)

In this chapter I shall present an account of some individual weekly psychotherapeutic work with a single mother who first presented to the clinic as a parent seeking help for herself and one of her sons. This case is therefore an example of a particular group of cases in which a parent may be offered therapy in their own right, appropriately in my view, within a CAMH service. There are also cases where work with the parental couple would in a similar way be the outcome of an exploration of who it is in a family who needs to be offered treatment. This approach runs counter to an emphasis on the named patient (the child or adolescent) as the primary patient.

The patient I shall describe is a 54-year-old woman. Important in her story as it unfolds in the here-and-now of the therapy are her two sons: the older one, Don, is 26, the younger Tobias is 14. My patient rang up the clinic about a year ago, asking for help for herself and her younger son in coping with Don's schizophrenic breakdown. I first saw Mrs C and Tobias together for an exploratory interview. At that time, they were both very frightened and confused about what was happening to Don, and under particular stress because Don thought that he was quite rational and that it was the people who were worried about him who were ill. There was palpable relief during the initial consultation when I spoke about their anger and when Tobias made it clear that he would like some of the burdensome responsibility of supporting his mother to be shifted from his shoulders to mine. In the initial period of work, I then saw Mrs C and Tobias separately a couple of times, and after that offered to see her fortnightly on a short-term basis with a focus on helping her to sort out how she could cope both with Don's collapse, and his massive demands on her, and find a way to protect Tobias, whose day-to-day life was in danger of being taken over by his half-brother's psychosis. How to mother both sons was the problem for which she wanted help at this point.

Within a short period of beginning work with me, and following Don's having voluntarily accepted psychiatric intervention, her own depression and anxiety began to flood into our sessions. Less and less was she able to summon the adult part of her personality to think with me about the management of this family crisis. It became quite clear that she felt herself in urgent need of psychotherapy and it became possible for me to offer this a few months later.

Here briefly is the story of her life as it emerged in the early sessions. She is the eldest of three daughters born to an English clergyman serving with the British Army in India and his wife, who later became a successful academic. She spent the first four years of her life in India cared for by a succession of Indian ayahs, and was then placed in a boarding school in England. Her memories of her parents are dominated by a picture of a very cold, hostile, angry marriage, of very harsh and demanding expectations of the children, enforced by severe discipline, all of this served up as good for their souls. There seem to be no memories of being understood, but a pervasive feeling of trying to find out how to avoid being in the wrong, interspersed with occasional rebellious moments when being a bad girl seemed to be the only way she could live. She remained at boarding schools when her parents eventually returned to live in England. She was not seen as academically capable, and everyone seemed surprised by her good results in exams. The family opposed her wish to go to art school, and she settled for training as a nursery teacher. She was very successful in this profession, at one time owning her own school, and she greatly liked working with young children.

In her late 20s, one of the moments of rebellion took told of her: she conceived a child by a man with whom the relationship ended almost immediately. Her family summoned the full weight of the authority of church and medicine to persuade her to have an abortion, but she refused, believing that it was absolutely critical for her to give birth to this child. She was supported by one friend, who was an artist. Together they lived for a while in a hill village on a

Mediterranean island, where they reconstructed a collapsed house – Mrs C retains this house and spends holidays there. This baby was Don. Later, she returned to England and resumed teaching. She feels that Don had an extremely happy childhood. She was determined to give him all the intimacy and affection she herself had lacked, and he was a vigorous, imaginative and intelligent little boy who was very successful at school and in social relationships. When Don was ten, she met and married Sammy, an Afro-Caribbean man of great charm and social and political idealism. Tobias is their child. There was however a painful clash of expectations in this marriage: Sammy wanted his political activities to be backed by her full-time work and did not expect to give up his numerous relationships with other women. Eventually, when she returned home from her hospital stay after giving birth to Tobias to find another woman had moved into her flat, she realized that the relationship was intolerable to her. Sammy finally moved out. They have remained friends, and he is spasmodically and passionately involved with Tobias.

After the breakdown of the marriage, Mrs C developed breast cancer and had a mastectomy. Two years later there was a recurrence in the second breast. She was given a date for a second mastectomy. Over a period of ten days while waiting for this operation, a psychological crisis overtook her. She was sleepless, preoccupied with a vision of the interior of her body, 'seeing' in her mind's eye the cancer, and fighting it, making it die. She seems to have discovered quite on her own the process of visualization which subsequently became an established if unorthodox approach to cancer treatment. When she was admitted to hospital and the breast opened up, the cancerous lump had gone, shrunk to tiny dry remnants to the astonishment of her surgeon.

These events occurred five years before I met her. She was aware that although from one perspective she had won a battle with a life-threatening illness, she herself felt that her life had from her point of view ended then. When I saw her, she was very depressed in an underlying way, visible in her stooped, prematurely aged demeanour, in her shapeless jumble-sale clothes, her lifeless skin and hair. While her body thus spoke of one reality, her external life was a complex picture. She had been too depressed to return to work and was living on benefits, supplemented by small earnings. She had not been able to imagine any further relationship with a man. However, she functioned as a considerable resource in her neighbourhood where she edited the community magazine, was the secretary of the large communal garden and a source of wisdom, support and good sense to many individuals. While Don remained crippled by his illness, Tobias, despite the considerable strain he was under, was an outstandingly lively, attractive boy, with a very close relationship with his mother. It was as if Mrs C was now living for others, who were indeed benefitting from her love, while seeing her own personal life as ended. This was represented in her inability to write or paint, activities which had been earlier sources of pleasure to her.

Clinical material

She began this session with a reference to the mild anti-depressants her GP had prescribed, which had lifted the edge of her depression, so that she no longer felt 'down a hole,' and enabled her to sleep, though without dreaming. She said she felt this was all a bit of a cheat. I asked her about this idea of cheating or being cheated, and she replied that something was being avoided. I wondered whether this was linked with her mentioning the absence of dreams, and she said, "Yes, though actually I did have a dream about four nights ago. I dreamt that Nina was getting married. Tobias and I were feeling upset and hurt because we had not been invited to the wedding." She explained to me that Nina was the daughter of an old friend, and also a friend of Tobias's. These two look like twins in fact, both having white mothers and black fathers. Nina's father was Jamaican though he left before she was born. She went on,

> Nina used to be very close to me when she was a little girl because I was her nursery school teacher. She used to like to come home with me and play at doing my hair. I had a box of ribbons and another of clips, slides, and so on and she would like to play this for hours. Nina's own hair is coarse, Afro-hair, very difficult to care for.

I asked if she herself had any thoughts about this dream. She replied that she felt Nina might be an aspect of herself. I asked what she thought about her not being invited to the wedding. After a pause, she said that she thought Nina was going to marry a white man. It was not Nina's fault that they had not been asked. In the dream it was as if Mrs C was somehow ignoring the wedding. I linked this to the theme of cheating: what was being ignored in the dream seemed to be something of great emotional significance, like a wedding. "Yes," she replied. "I have been very busy all week preparing the room in my flat to let, which is a lot of work, and yesterday I spent the whole day catching up on my job as secretary of our communal garden." I spoke about her feeling aware of being very active but not allowing any time for thinking. There followed some talk of a visit from Sammy, and her quite new realization that she was no longer in love with him and some observations of Sammy's abrasive relationship with Don, whom he regards as a cop-out. She reported saying to Don, "There is no need for you to feel in rivalry with Sammy." I linked this to the dream: she and Tobias were upset about a wedding they felt excluded from, and now she was thinking about Don's upset about her marriage to Sammy, which she felt had made him feel excluded. She said, "Yes! Don says the main thing he has talked about in the first weeks of his therapy (this has been recently arranged) is his relationship with Sammy and how awful it was."

After a silence I said that in her dream she thought Nina was going to marry a white man, while she and Nina's mother had chosen black men. I wondered about this and said to her, "There is something important about these black and white skins for you." "Oh!" she shuddered, with a long intake of breath and trembling, taking time to gather her words. "Yes," she said. After quite a pause, she continued,

> Of course I was born in India. The first thing I was attracted to was the life of our Indian cook and his family, in the kitchen and beyond. But it was all forbidden territory to me. And I had Indian ayahs, lots of them. I can't remember a person's face at all; they changed all the time, because of rows with my mother. I remember one row, with my ayah crying, obviously having got the sack, and my mother shouting.

She spoke at length about the house (a large colonial bungalow), contrasting the cold atmosphere of her area – "all prohibitions and being smacked" – with the imagined delights of the kitchen. When I began to link together the feeling of all the warmth, food and comfort being with the servants, she interrupted me (a very unusual boldness for her!) and said, "But I wasn't allowed to have it. It was forbidden. All my life I've wanted to be accepted by black people, to

231

be a part of their lives." She also linked this with her father's family history – his family, from Liverpool, had a lot of money at one time. He had researched where this fortune had come from and was sure that it was based on involvement in the slave trade. Here surely was the forbidden and complicated background to her feeling of powerful attraction to relationships with black people.

She went on to connect these wishes with the hopes of her marriage, and spoke of the disappointments she endured, particularly all the things Sammy would not talk about.

There is much to explore in these associations, but I now want to add an important fact about this session which I was not able to make use of at the time. I myself was having two experiences in addition to the conversation I have reported. I was struggling with a frustrating conviction that I could not properly get hold of the transference situation in the session (what exactly was it that was being avoided in the ignoring of the marriage in the dream? What evasion of coming close to intense emotional experience?). Much more uncomfortable than this intellectual frustration was a state of irritable anxiety which was building up in me, particularly experienced as an urgent desire to suck or bite my fingers. My task was to work through these feelings and impulses, to work through this intense, disturbing countertransference reaction (Brenman Pick, 1985) and to make sense of it.

In the following session, the meaning of this projection began to emerge. Mrs C began by talking at length about Don, a story conveying a complex mixture – he has done lots of work (he is a capable carpenter and joiner), they have had some really good talks as they have not done for years, and he has re-established his links with old friends. On the other hand, although he acknowledges he is an alcoholic, he has been drinking very heavily, and then he oversleeps for hours which makes Tobias very angry. Tobias finds and confiscates his half empty bottles of whiskey, and is furious that Don is sleeping all these extra hours – he wants Don to go back to his own flat. She went on to reveal that Don steals drink from her, including her specially kept homemade wine, and to puzzle about why she cannot confront him about the £5 a week he has agreed to pay for food but never remembers to give her.

I found myself plagued by similar surges of anxious discomfort to those of last week's session while she was speaking. I explored the financial arrangements with her and we established that £5 was a very unrealistically low sum for Don to pay for his food. She reflected again on her perception of him as a small boy, and her feeling that she needed to allow him to be so, in contrast with her anger about his stealing from her. She described a real fury at finding the homemade wine nearly all gone. "Why is it so hard for me to ask him for money?" she asked. I talked about her seeing Don as a baby who has not yet grasped that he does not possess all of mother as a right: she seems in part to agree with Don that everything that she has is automatically his, although another part of her is furious and sees this as greedy exploitation and dishonesty. But this part of her seems located in Tobias, who voices it very clearly. She assented and described how when Don was sitting there with his thumb in his mouth saying seductively how absolutely delicious her ginger wine was, she felt enraged but also overwhelmed.

At this moment, I felt the relief of illumination. The image of Don with his thumb in his mouth linked with my impulse to suck and chew my fingers during these last two sessions, an impulse which I felt was being irresistibly projected into me. Now I thought I knew where this was coming from. So I gathered the threads I could now follow. I reminded her that last week we spoke about her first childhood home and the kitchen which she felt was the source of real life and warmth which she was excluded from. I described to her a little girl part of herself that felt and is still feeling unbearable deprivation about being shut out of that place, and confined to what felt like the emotionally cold part of the house and the harshness of her parents. Now, when she indulges Don's sense of need and deprivation, she is feeding the unhappy little girl in herself, who has felt a lifelong deprivation and emptiness in her mouth. "Oh . . . Oh I see . . . I see . . ." she whispered in anguish and then wept. "Poor Don." I spoke about the regret and concern she was feeling about the use she has made of Don, but suggested that she was again at this moment putting into him the painful sense of emptiness and thus feeling sympathy for him. . . . "Instead of myself," she said thus finishing the sentence herself. "Yes." "Do I do it to Tobias too?" she asked anxiously. I reminded her that earlier she was telling me that Tobias had to bear the anger, the sense that there was something about Don's behaviour that needed to be dealt with, something to put a stop to.

She then spoke at length about many people over the years telling her that she was too close to Don and her knowing there was something in this idea but never understanding what it was. She cried for quite a while and I wondered with her if the tears expressed not only some relief and gratitude for understanding something, but also a complaint to me that this getting-to-know herself was too painful, that I had hurt her too much. "No," she said. "It is like having a boil lanced."

Later, at the end of the session she said that she thought she has never been able to be fully inside herself. "This leaking of feelings has always happened, hasn't it? Does awareness of it make it possible to stop the leaks?"

Discussion

In these sessions, I think the projections into her children and into me in the transference are fairly transparent. I registered for her, for example, the aching emptiness and rage of her baby self faced with the vision of unattainable plenitude, and the scepticism of her adult self about Don's relative poverty and the need to placate and indulge his greed. I also functioned for her as a person capable of thinking over time, waiting for links to become clearer, tolerating the discomfort or uncertainty. There is also evidence when she wonders about her leakiness that she takes in this idea that thinking about states of mind might make a difference. I think at that moment she experienced a potential identification with what I had been doing in the session. With shock and pain, but also relief and a clearer sense that there could be a place inside herself where she could feel contained, a mental space, she took hold of the anger projected into Tobias and the possessive and delinquent greed and confusion so manifest in Don.

Further clinical material

I now want to describe a brief sequence from a session two weeks later. The earlier part of the session had dealt with Mrs C's sense of herself as a child dependent on powerful authorities who were in overt and covert conflict with each other: the child therefore did not know where to put herself since any alliance had dangerous consequences. Historically this referred to her quarrelling parents, resurrected in the present in the conflicting views in the medical profession about the correct approach to her son's schizophrenia, and in her confusion about whether the antidepressants her GP had prescribed for her might actually attack her capacity to work with me in therapy. She then mentioned the strange state of mind she had been in for the last few days. When I asked her to tell me more about this, after a thoughtful pause she began to talk about being in Waitrose (a supermarket close to the Clinic) on Saturday. It was rather crowded. She was standing in one of those long queues waiting. As she stood there, she found herself thinking, "Matter is only energy . . . so there is really no reason why I cannot be transformed into pure energy, and float past the queue and the till and through the plate glass window. It seemed perfectly possible."

At this point in the session, the transference situation became clear to me, so I said to her that I thought the context of these thoughts could help us to understand what is happening inside her. She is describing to me a setting in which she is faced with a frustrating, maybe also irritating wait in a queue, in order to acquire what she needs to sustain life, the food she wants to buy from Waitrose. But perhaps this also represents the therapy – the food for thought for which she comes to see me. We have been talking about the session I have to cancel soon and the Easter holiday which comes after that, and I think she is telling me that this feels a very concrete experience for her; access to me feels overcrowded, getting what she wants from me is now dominated by images of having to wait. What seems to happen is that she imagines being able to slip out of her place in the queue and evade all the frustration and perhaps anger that being there involves. Drifting out of her skin, she seems to acquire in fantasy what she wants without having to ask or acknowledge anyone else, and without having to pay the price. The price asked here involves her enduring feelings of disappointment and anger. In her fantasy all boundaries dissolve, like the plate glass window. In her mind she is dissolving the upsetting facts of reality, the session she will miss, the coming holiday break and indeed the closeness now to the ending of today's session.

"That is *exactly* how I feel," she said. "You are quite right."

I added that she was wondering whether I was as frightened of her anger as she was. It was interesting that when she left the room she offered none of the thank-yous or other appreciative remarks she usually made. The session-end had a much sharper edge in consequence.

Mrs C is now becoming more able to have and to hold on to her experience of feeling excluded, made to wait and made aware of all the others in the queue, the many competitors she feels stand in the way of her being attended to. We see vividly the depletion of her psychic resources which resulted from the massive splitting of her personality and the strengthening effect, making her more solid and real, of the regained contact with her infantile anger and rage.

Thinking for oneself

An interesting image was introduced by the patient at the end of the following session. She found herself thinking about the plants on her veranda and told me that she grows many plants there, and also inside her flat. She was imagining a plant being cut back from a spindly overgrown luxuriance to allow for the development of a more solid stem. She explained that this wild growth was like a picture of how she had lived in the earlier part of her adult life. She had sprouted many long tendrils, but she had to attach herself to a trellis for support to hold up this over-grown state. Sammy was like this trellis for her for some while. But now something different is happening – this wild growth is being replaced by growth from the roots. It is to do with coming here and thinking about growing older, and where she wants to be, and being able to let go of Don and Tobias, and to be on her own. There is something she likes very much about being able to be alone. She developed this thought in relation to plans for her summer holiday and talked about being able to walk alone along the seashore, and watch the mermaids. "That is where I want to be," she said. I replied that she wanted to be in a place where she could hear her own thoughts and feelings and imaginings, and that she was also letting me go and acknowledging being alone without her session next week.

In this sequence, my patient is sharing with me the growth of her thinking and her powers of self-observation, and telling me how she has become interested in herself. She describes the experience of me as the gardener able to differentiate healthy and unhealthy growth, to show her that the spindly attachments to the trellis of her relationships involve an entwining with the trellis which weakens her own identity. The cutting-back is an image of the withdrawal of massive and very extensive projections and the concentration of growing effort in the stalk of the plant-baby we are taking care of together in therapy.

The psychoanalytic process which is taking place in our relationship has opened up a re-connection with her roots. One might indeed wonder whether I am linked in her mind with the gardener of her childhood home (she had described the huge garden lovingly), and in the present her place with me in therapy is providing her with the possibility of stronger growth. The imagery she uses is extraordinarily apt for her physical being – she is a very tall woman, rather like a gangly teenager in her long limbs, but her stoop conveys well the weakened backbone of her psychic state.

To evade the miseries of her anxious and hostile attachment to her internal parents, she seems to have retreated to a very primitive adhesive attachment to the emotionally significant others of her world when she felt that clinging to them was life-saving. This sticky attachment has to be relinquished, the other has to be allowed to be separate, before she can take in the potential for her own separate hold on life. Esther Bick (1968, 1986) has written of this primitive adhesive identification in infantile psychic life which persists when there is no adequate container available for the intense infantile anxieties. My patient's courage when she is offered in the transference relationship maternal containment for her infantile anxieties is extremely impressive. One is reminded of her self-cure from the second cancer. This unusual capacity to make use of her therapist speaks to a part of herself that has remained alive, trying to find what she needed throughout her life. Her choice of profession kept her in touch with young children externally and with that part of herself internally.

I will conclude by differentiating three kinds of interpretations in my work with her. My central focus was on describing the relationship she made with me. This is the transference core, sometimes plainly evident as in the material about the plants and the supermarket. The point of interpreting this is to give her access to the nature of her internal world and thus potential freedom from unconscious determination of her relationships. With this patient, who has become close to her inner preoccupations in the course of therapy (when she began, she spoke only of others, never of herself, never of 'I'), there is also much work on describing the different parts of herself and exploring their internal relationship. For example, her identification with the primitive parents at the expense of the needy little girl self, which became painfully evident when she described a whole day of working and not eating till 9.30 p.m. at night, and not realizing why she was feeling so ill. Lastly, there is the scrutiny of my countertransference experience, which provides clues to the meaning of her associations. My task is to work over in my mind precisely what she has not been able to digest, to the point where I can see a way of helping her to take back into herself what she first needed to lodge in me.

References

Ali, M. (2003) *Brick Lane*. London: Doubleday.

Alvarez, A. (1992) *Live Company: Psychoanalytic Psychotherapy with Autistic, Borderline, Deprived and Abused Children*. London: Routledge.

Alvarez, A. and Reid, S. (eds.) (1999) *Autism and Personality: Findings from the Tavistock Autism Workshop*. London: Routledge.

Bailey, T. (2006) 'There's no such thing as an adolescent'. In: M. Lanyado and A. Horne (eds.) *A Question of Technique: Independent Psychoanalytic Approaches with Children and Adolescents*. London: Routledge.

Barrows, P. (1995) 'Oedipal issues at 4 and 44'. *Psychoanalytic Psychotherapy*, 9 (1): 85–96.

Bick, E. (1964) 'Notes on infant observation in psycho-analytic training'. *International Journal of Psychoanalysis*, 45: 558–566.

Bick, E. (1968) 'The experience of the skin in early object relations'. *International Journal of Psychoanalysis*, 49: 484–486.

Bick, E. (1986) 'Further considerations on the function of the skin in early object relations: Findings from infant observation integrated into child and adult analysis'. *British Journal of Psychotherapy*, 2 (4): 292–299.

Bion, W. R. (1957) 'Differentiation of the psychotic from the non-psychotic personalities'. *International Journal of Psychoanalysis*, 38: 206–275.

Bion, W. R. (1959) 'Attacks on linking'. *International Journal of Psychoanalysis*, 40: 308–315. Reprinted in W. R. Bion: *Second Thoughts: Selected Papers on Psychoanalysis.*. London: Heinemann, 1967.

Bion, W. R. (1962a) *Learning from Experience*. London: Tavistock Publications. Republished Maresfield Reprints, 1984.

Bion, W. R. (1962b) 'A theory of thinking'. *International Journal of Psychoanalysis*, 43: 306–310. Reprinted in W. R. Bion: *Second Thoughts: Selected Papers on Psychoanalysis*. London: Heinemann, 1967.

Bion, W. R. (1970) *Attention and Interpretation*. London: Tavistock Publications.

Bion, W. R. (1976 [1994]) 'Emotional turbulence'. In: F. Bion (ed.) *Clinical Seminars and Other Works*. London: Karnac.

Bion, W. R. (1979 [1994]) 'Making the best of a bad job'. In: F. Bion (ed.) *Clinical Seminars and Other Works*. London: Karnac.

Birksted-Breen, D. (1996) 'Phallus, penis and mental space'. *International Journal of Psychoanalysis*, 77 (4): 649–657.

Boston, M. (1972) 'Psychotherapy with a boy from a children's home'. *Journal of Child Psychotherapy*, 3: 53–67.

Boston, M., Lush, D. and Grainger, E. (1991) 'Evaluation of psychoanalytic psychotherapy with children: Therapists' assessments and predictions'. *Psychoanalytic Psychotherapy*, 5 (3): 191–234.

Boston, M. and Szur, R. (eds.) (1983) *Psychotherapy with Severely Deprived Children*. London: Routledge.

Britton, R. (1981) 'Re-enactment as an unwitting professional response to family dynamics'. In: S. Box, B. Copley, J. Magagna and E. Moustaki (eds.) *Psychotherapy with Families: An Analytic Approach*. London: Routledge.

Britton, R. (1983) 'Breakdown and reconstitution of the family circle'. In: M. Boston and R. Szur (eds.) *Psychotherapy with Severely Deprived Children*. London: Routledge.

Britton, R. (1989) 'The missing link: Parental sexuality and the Oedipus complex'. In: J. Steiner (ed.) *The Oedipus Complex Today: Clinical Implications*. London: Karnac.

Britton, R. (1998) *Belief and Imagination: Explorations in Psychoanalysis*. London: Routledge, New Library of Psychoanalysis.

Canham, H. (1999) 'The development of the concept of time in fostered and adopted children'. *Psychoanalytic Inquiry*, 19 (2): 160–171.

Copley, B. (1987) 'Explorations with families'. *Journal of Child Psychotherapy*, 13 (1): 93–108.

Cregeen, S. (2009) 'Exposed: Phallic protections, shame and damaged parental objects'. *Journal of Child Psychotherapy*, 35 (1): 32–48.

Cregeen, S. (2017) 'A place within the heart: Finding a home with parental objects'. *Journal of Child Psychotherapy*, 43 (2): 159–174.

Cregeen, S., Hughes, C., Midgley, N., Rhode, M. and Rustin, M. (2017) *Short-Term Psychoanalytic Psychotherapy for Adolescents with Depression: A Treatment Manual*. London: Karnac.

Dartington, A. (1998) 'The intensity of adolescence in small families'. In: R. Anderson and A. Dartington (eds.) *Facing It Out: Clinical Perspectives on Adolescent Disturbance*. London: Duckworth.

Daws, D. (1989) *Through the Night: Helping Parents and Sleepless Infants*. London: Free Association Books.

Department of Health (2003) *Getting the Right Start: National Service Framework for Children: Emerging Findings*. London: Department of Health.

Dockar-Drysdale, B. (1990) *The Provision of Primary Experience: Winnicottian Work with Children and Adolescents*. London: Free Association Books.

Emanuel, R. (1984) 'Primary disappointment'. *Journal of Child Psychotherapy*, 10: 71–87.

Etchegoyen, A. (1997) 'Inhibition of mourning and the replacement child syndrome'. In: J. Raphael-Leff and R. J. Perelberg (eds.) *Female Experience: Three Generations of British Women Psychoanalysts on Work with Women*. London: Routledge.

Freud, S. (1917 [1915]) 'Mourning and melancholia'. In: *The Standard Edition of the Complete Psychological Works of Sigmund Freud* (vol. 14, pp. 237–258). London: Hogarth.

Furniss, T. (1991) *The Multiprofessional Handbook of Child Sexual Abuse: Integrated Management, Therapy, and Legal Intervention*. London: Routledge.

Goodyer, I. M., Reynolds, S., Barrett, B., Byford, S., Dubicka, B., Hill, J., Holland, F., Kelvin, R., Midgley, N., Roberts, C., Senior, R., Target, M., Widmer, B., Wilkinson, P. and Fonagy, P. (2017) 'Cognitive behavioural therapy and short-term psychoanalytical psychotherapy versus a brief psychosocial intervention in adolescents with unipolar major depressive disorder (IMPACT): A multicentre, pragmatic, observer-blind, randomised controlled superiority trial'. *Lancet*, 4 (2): 109–119.

Gretton, A. (2006) 'An account of a year's work with a mother and her 18-month-old son at risk of autism'. *International Journal of Infant Observation*, 9 (1): 21–34.

Harris, M. (1966) 'Therapeutic Consultations'. *Journal of Child Psychotherapy*, 1 (4): 13–19. Reprinted in M. Harris Williams (ed.) *The Tavistock Model: Collected Papers of Martha Harris and Esther Bick*. Strath Tay: Clunie Press, 1987.

Harris, M. (1968) 'The child psychotherapist and the patient's family'. *Journal of Child Psychotherapy*, 2 (2): 50–63.

Harris, M. (1975) 'Some notes on maternal containment in "good enough" mothering'. *Journal of Child Psychotherapy*, 4 (1): 35–51.

Harris, M. and Meltzer, D. (1976) 'A psychoanalytic model of the child-in-the-family-in-the-community'. OECD report reprinted in: A. Hahn (ed.) *Sincerity and Other Works: Collected Papers of Donald Meltzer*. London: Karnac, 1994.

Harris, M. and Meltzer, D. (1986) 'Family patterns and cultural educability'. In: D. Meltzer (ed.) *Studies in Extended Metapsychology: Clinical Applications of Bion's Ideas*. Strath Tay: Clunie Press.

Henry, G. (1974) 'Doubly deprived'. *Journal of Child Psychotherapy*, 3 (4): 15–28.

Hindle, D. (2000) 'An intensive assessment of a small sample of siblings placed together in foster care'. Unpublished Tavistock/University of East London Prof Doc thesis.

Hodges, J. and Steele, M. (1995) 'Internal representations of parent–child attachments in maltreated children'. Paper presented to the Thomas Coran Foundation Conference 'New Developments in Attachment Theory', September.

Hoffman, E. (1989) *Lost in Translation: A Life in a New Language.* New York: Penguin.

Hopkins, J. (1992) 'Infant-parent psychotherapy'. *Journal of Child Psychotherapy*, 18 (1): 5–17.

Houzel, D. (2001) 'Bisexual qualities of the psychic envelope'. In: J. Edwards (ed.) *Being Alive: Building on the work of Anne Alvarez.* Hove: Brunner-Routledge.

Isaacs, S. (1948) 'On the nature and function of phantasy'. *International Journal of Psychoanalysis*, 29: 73–97. Republished in: M. Klein, P. Heimann, S. Isaacs and J. Riviere (eds.) *Developments in Psycho-Analysis.* London: Hogarth, 1952.

Kennedy, E. (2003) *Child and Adolescent Psychotherapy: A Systematic Review of Psychoanalytic Approaches.* London: North Central London Strategic Health Authority.

Kennedy, E. and Midgley, N. (eds.) (2007) *Process and Outcome Research in Child Adolescent and Parent-Infant Psychotherapy: A Thematic Review.* London: NHS London.

Klauber, T. (1998) 'The significance of trauma in work with the parents of severely disturbed children, and its implications for work with parents in general'. *Journal of Child Psychotherapy*, 24 (1): 85–107.

Klein, M. (1935) 'A Contribution to the Psychogenesis of Manic-Depressive States'. In: *Love, Guilt and Reparation and Other Works 1921–1945 (The Writings of Melanie Klein, Volume 1).* London: Hogarth Press. [Reprinted London: Vintage, 1988].

Klein, M. (1936) 'Weaning'. In: *Love, Guilt and Reparation and Other Works 1921-1945 (The Writings of Melanie Klein, Volume 1).* London: Hogarth Press. [Reprinted London: Vintage, 1988].

Klein, M. (1940) 'Mourning and its relation to manic-depressive states'. In: *Love, Guilt and Reparation and Other Works 1921–1945 (The Writings of Melanie Klein, Volume 1).* London: Hogarth Press. [Reprinted London: Vintage, 1988].

Klein, M. (1945) 'The Oedipus Complex in the light of early anxieties'. In: *Love, Guilt and Reparation and Other Works 1921–1945 (The Writings of Melanie Klein, Volume 1).* London: Hogarth Press. [Reprinted London: Vintage, 1988].

Klein, M. (1946) 'Notes on some schizoid mechanisms'. In: *Envy and Gratitude and Other Works 1946–1963 (1975) (The Writings of Melanie Klein, Volume 3)*. London: Hogarth. [Reprinted London: Vintage, 1997].

Kraemer, S. (1997) 'What narrative?'. In: R. Papadopoulos and J. Byng-Hall (eds.) *Multiple Voices: Narrative in Systemic Family Psychotherapy*. London: Duckworth.

Levi, P. (1958) *If This Is A Man*. Harmondsworth: Penguin.

Lindsey, C. (1997) 'New stories for old? The creation of new families by adoption and fostering'. In: R. Papadopoulos and J. Byng-Hall (eds.) *Multiple Voices: Narrative in Systemic Family Psychotherapy*. London: Duckworth.

Malloch, S. and Trevarthen, C. (eds.) (2009) *Communicative Musicality: Exploring the Basis of Human Companionship*. Oxford: Oxford University Press.

Meltzer, D. (1967) *The Psychoanalytic Process*. London: Heinemann.

Meltzer, D. (1981) 'The Kleinian expansion of Freud's metapsychology'. *International Journal of Psychoanalysis*, 62 (2): 177–185.

Miller, L. (1992) 'The relation of infant observation to clinical practice in an under-fives counselling service'. *Journal of Child Psychotherapy*, 18 (1): 19–32.

Money-Kyrle, R. E. (1968) 'Cognitive development'. *International Journal of Psychoanalysis*, 49 (2): 691–698.

Morgan, M. (2019) *A Couple State of Mind: Psychoanalysis of Couples and the Tavistock Relationships Model*. Abingdon: Routledge.

O'Shaughnessy, E. (1989) 'The invisible Oedipus complex'. In: R. Britton, M. Feldman, E. O'Shaughnessy, H. Segal and J. Steiner (eds.) *The Oedipus Complex Today: Clinical Implications*. London: Karnac.

Pick, I. B. (1985) 'Working through in the countertransference'. *International Journal of Psychoanalysis*, 66 (2): 157–166.

Reid, S. (1999a) 'The assessment of the child with autism: A family perspective'. In: A. Alvarez and S. Reid (eds.) *Autism and Personality: Findings from the Tavistock Autism Workshop*. London: Routledge.

Reid, S. (1999b) 'The group as a healing whole: Group psychotherapy with children and adolescents'. In: M. Lanyado and A. Horn (eds.) *The Handbook of Child and Adolescent Psychotherapy*. London: Routledge.

Rhode, M. (2008) 'Joining the human family'. In: K. Barrows (ed.) *Autism in Childhood and Autistic Features in Adults*. London: Karnac.

Rosenberg, E. B. (1992) *The Adoption Life Cycle: The Children and their Families through the Years*. New York: Free Press.

Rustin, M. E. (2001) 'The therapist with her back against the wall'. *Journal of Child Psychotherapy*, 27 (3): 273–284.

Rustin, M. E. (2006) 'Where do I belong? Dilemmas for children and adolescents who have been adopted or brought up in long-term foster care'. In: J. Kenrick, C. Lindsey and L. Tollemache (eds.) *Creating New Families: Therapeutic Approaches to Fostering, Adoption, and Kinship Care*. London: Karnac.

Rustin, M. E. (2009) 'Esther Bick's legacy of infant observation at the Tavistock: Some reflections 60 years on'. *International Journal of Infant Observation*, 12 (1): 29–41.

Rustin, M. E. (2016) 'Infant observation: A method of psychoanalytic learning and an influence on clinical practice'. In: A. Elliott and J. Prager (eds.) *The Routledge Handbook of Psychoanalysis in the Social Sciences and Humanities*. London: Routledge.

Rustin, M. E. and Rustin, M. J. (eds.) (2019) *New Discoveries in Child Psychotherapy: Findings from Qualitative Research*. London: Routledge.

Rustin, M. J., Rustin, M. E., Anderson, J., Cohn, N., Hindle, D., Ironside, L. and Philps, J. (2003) 'Borderline Organisations'. Paper given at conference of Tavistock Society of Psychotherapists.

Segal, H. (1957) 'Notes on symbol formation'. *International Journal of Psychoanalysis*, 38: 391–397.

Shribman, S. (2007) *Children's Health, Our Future. A Review of Progress against the National Service Framework for Children, Young People and Maternity Services 2004*. London: Department of Health.

Shuttleworth, A. (1982) 'Finding a way to the parent'. Unpublished paper given at the Inter-Clinic Conference in October 1982 as part of a Tavistock Clinic contribution on 'Concepts of Change'.

Sorensen, P. B. (1997) 'Thoughts on the containing process from the perspective of infant/mother relations'. In: S. Reid (ed.) *Developments in Infant Observation: The Tavistock Model*. London: Routledge.

The Stationery Office (2003) *The Victoria Climbié Inquiry Report*. London: The Stationery Office.

Steiner, J. (1985) 'Turning a blind eye: The cover up for Oedipus'. *International Review of Psychoanalysis*, 12: 161–172.

Steiner, J. (1993) *Psychic Retreats: Pathological Organizations in Psychotic, Neurotic and Borderline Patients*. London: Routledge.

Summit, R. C. (1983) 'The child sexual abuse accommodation syndrome'. *Child Abuse and Neglect*, 7 (2): 177–193.

Tanner, K. (1999) 'Observation: A counter culture offensive. Observation's contribution to the development of reflective social work practice'. *International Journal of Infant Observation*, 2 (2): 12–32.

Tischler, S. (1979) 'Being with a psychotic child: A psychoanalytical approach to the problems of parents of psychotic children'. *International Journal of Psychoanalysis*, 60 (1): 29–38.

Trowell, J. and Etchegoyen, A. (2002) *The Importance of Fathers: A Psycho-analytic Re-Evaluation*. London: Routledge.

Trowell, J., Joffe, I., Campbell, J., Clemente, C., Almqvist, F., Soininen, M., Koskenranta-Aalto, U., Weintraub, S., Kolaitis, G., Tomaras, V., Anastasopoulis, D., Grayson, K., Barnes, J. and Tsiantis, J. (2007) 'Childhood depression: A place for psychotherapy'. *European Child and Adolescent Psychiatry* 16 (3): 157–167.

Tsiantis, J. (ed.) (1999) *Working with Parents of Children and Adolescents Who Are in Psychoanalytic Psychotherapy*, EFPP Clinical Monograph. London: Karnac.

Tustin, F. (1981) *Autistic States in Children*. London: Routledge and Kegan Paul.

Waddell, M. (1998) *Inside Lives: Psychoanalysis and the Growth of the Personality*. London: Duckworth.

Winnicott, D. W. (1971) *Therapeutic Consultations in Child Psychiatry*. London: Hogarth and Institute of Psycho-Analysis.

Youell, B. (1999) 'From observation to working with a child'. *International Journal of Infant Observation*, 2 (2): 78–90.

Margaret Rustin publications 1971–2020

Books

Understanding Your Nine Year Old (with E. O'Shaughnessy). Corgi, 1972.

Narratives of Love and Loss: Studies in Modern Children's Fiction (with Michael Rustin). Verso, 1987.

Closely Observed Infants (co-editor with L. Miller, Michael Rustin and J. Shuttleworth). Duckworth, 1989.

Psychotic States in Children (co-editor with A. Dubinsky, H. Dubinsky and M. Rhode). (Tavistock Clinic Series). Duckworth, 1997.

Assessment in Child Psychotherapy (co-editor with E. Quagliata) (Tavistock Clinic Series). Karnac, 1997.

Mirror to Nature: Drama, Psychoanalysis and Society (with Michael Rustin). (Tavistock Clinic Series). Karnac, 2002.

Work Discussion: Learning from Reflective Practice in Work with Children and Families (co-editor with J. Bradley). (Tavistock Clinic Series). Karnac, 2008.

Enabling and Inspiring: A Tribute to Martha Harris (co-editor with M. Harris Williams, M. Rhode and G. Williams). Karnac, 2012.

Young Child Observation: A Development in the Theory and Method of Infant Observation (co-editor with S. M. G. Adamo). (Tavistock Clinic Series). Karnac, 2013.

Reading Klein (with Michael Rustin) (New Library of Psychoanalysis Teaching Series). Routledge, 2016.

Short-Term Psychoanalytic Psychotherapy for Adolescents with Depression: A Treatment Manual (with S. Cregeen, C. Hughes, N. Midgley, M. Rhode, edited by J. Catty). (Tavistock Clinic Series). Karnac, 2016.

New Discoveries in Child Psychotherapy: Findings from Qualitative Research (with Michael Rustin). (Tavistock Clinic Series). Routledge, 2019.

Published papers/chapters in English

1971: Once-weekly work with a rebellious adolescent girl. *Journal of Child Psychotherapy*, 3 (1): 40–48.

1982: Finding a way to the child. *Journal of Child Psychotherapy*, 8 (2): 145–50.

1987: Encountering primitive anxieties: some aspects of infant observation as a preparation for clinical work with children and families. *Journal of Child Psychotherapy*, 14 (2): 15–28.

1991: The strengths of a practitioner's workshop as a new model in clinical research. In Szur, R. and Miller, S. (eds.) *Extending Horizons: Psychoanalytic Psychotherapy with Children, Adolescents and Families*. Karnac.

1994: (with Michael Rustin) Coups d'état and catastrophic change. *British Journal of Psychotherapy*, 11: 242–259.

1995: What follows family breakdown: the psychotherapeutic assessment of fostered and adopted children. In Quagliata, E. (ed.) *Un Buon Incontro*. Astrolabio.

1997: Child psychotherapy within the Kleinian tradition. In Burgoyne, B. and Sullivan, M. (eds.) *The Klein-Lacan Dialogues*. Karnac.

1998: Dialogues with parents. *Journal of Child Psychotherapy*, 24 (2): 233–252.

1998: Observation, understanding and interpretation: the story of a supervision. *Journal of Child Psychotherapy*, 24 (3): 433–448.

1999: Age. In: Taylor, D. (ed.) *Talking Cure: Mind and Method of the Tavistock Clinic*. Duckworth.

1999: Are children innocent? In: Taylor, D. (ed.) *Talking Cure: Mind and Method of the Tavistock Clinic*. Duckworth.

1999: Beginning of the mind. In: Taylor, D. (ed.) *Talking Cure: Mind and Method of the Tavistock Clinic*. Duckworth.

1999: Food for the mind. In: Taylor, D. (ed.) *Talking Cure: Mind and Method of the Tavistock Clinic*. Duckworth.

1999: Multiple families in mind: *Clinical Child Psychology and Psychiatry*, 4 (1): 51–62.

1999: The place of consultation with parents and therapy of parents in child psychotherapy. In Lanyado, M. and Horne, A. (eds.) *The Handbook of Child and Adolescent Psychotherapy: Psychoanalytic Approaches*. Routledge.

1999: The training of child psychotherapists at the Tavistock Clinic: philosophy and practice. *Psychoanalytic Inquiry*, 19: 125–141.

2000: Beckett: dramas of psychic catastrophe. In Cohen, M. and Hahn, A. (eds.) *Exploring the Work of Donald Meltzer: A Festschrift*. Karnac.

2001: Harry Potter's power to enchant. *Books for Keeps*, 130.

2001: The therapist with her back against the wall. *Journal of Child Psychotherapy*, 27 (3): 273–284.

2001 (with L.T. Buck): Thoughts on transitions between cultures: Jonathan moves from home to school and from class to class. *Infant Observation*, 4 (2): 121–133.

2002: Struggles in becoming a mother: reflections from a clinical and observational standpoint. *Infant Observation*, 5 (1): 7–20.

2002: (with R. Emanuel and L. Miller) Supervision of therapy of sexually abused girls. *Clinical Child Psychology and Psychiatry*, 7 (4): 581–594.

2003: (with R. Davenhill, A. Balfour, M. Blanchard, K. Tress) Looking into later life: psychodynamic observation and old age. *Psychoanalytic Psychotherapy*, 17 (3): 253–266.

2003: (with Michael Rustin) Where is home?: an essay on Philip Pullman's *Northern Lights*, Vol 1 of *His Dark Materials. Journal of Child Psychotherapy*, 29 (1): 93–105.

2003: (with Michael Rustin) A new kind of friendship: an essay on Philip Pullman's *The Subtle Knife*, Vol 2 of *His Dark Materials. Journal of Child Psychotherapy*, 29 (2): 227–241,

2003: (with Michael Rustin) Learning to say goodbye: an essay on Philip Pullman's *The Amber Spyglass*, Vol 3 of *His Dark Materials. Journal of Child Psychotherapy*, 29 (3): 415–428.

2004: Pullman's daemons. *Books for Keeps*, 145.

2004: Psychotherapy and community care. In: Rhode, M. and Klauber, T. (eds.) *The Many Faces of Asperger's Syndrome*. Karnac.

2005: Conceptual analysis of critical moments in Victoria Climbié's life. *Child & Family Social Work*, 10 (1): 11–19.

2005: (with Michael Rustin) Narratives and phantasies. In Vetere, A. and Dowling, E. (eds.) *Narrative Therapies with Children and their Families: A Practitioner's Guide to Concepts and Approaches*. Routledge.

2006: Where do I belong?: dilemmas for children and adolescents who have been adopted or brought up in long-term foster care. In: Kenrick, J., Lindsey, C. and Tollemache, L. (eds.) *Creating New Families: Therapeutic Approaches to Fostering, Adoption and Kinship Care*. Karnac.

2007: John Bowlby at the Tavistock. *Attachment and Human Development*, 9 (4): 355–359.

2007: Taking account of siblings: a view from child therapy. *Journal of Child Psychotherapy*, 33 (1): 21–25.

2008: The place of siblings in psychological development. In M. Klett-Davies (ed.) *Putting Siblings on the Map: A Multi-disciplinary Perspective*. Family and Parenting Institute.

2009: Esther Bick's legacy of infant observation at the Tavistock – some reflections 60 years on. *Infant Observation*, 12 (1): 29–41.

2009: (with B. Miller) Observation observed: closely observed infants on film. DVD-PAL. Tavistock & Portman NHS Trust.

2009: The psychology of depression in young adolescents: a psychoanalytic view of origins, inner workings and implications. *Psychoanalytic Psychotherapy*, 23 (3): 213–224.

2010: The complexities of service supervision: an experiential discovery. *Journal of Child Psychotherapy*, 36 (1): 3–15.

2010: (with L. Emanuel) Observation, reflection and containment: a psychoanalytic approach to work with parents and children under five. In A. Lemma and M. Patrick (eds.) *Off the Couch: Contemporary Psychoanalytic Applications*. Routledge.

2010: (with Michael Rustin) States of narcissism. In A. Varchevker and E. McGinley (eds.) *Enduring Loss: Mourning, Depression and Narcissism Throughout the Life Cycle*. Karnac.

2011: Passion in the classroom: understanding some vicissitudes in teacher-pupil relationships and the unavoidable anxieties of learning. In: Harris, R., Rendall, S. and Nashat, S. (eds.) *Engaging with Complexity: Child and Adolescent Mental Health and Education*. Routledge.

2012: Discussion of Rosemary Randall's chapter 'Great expectations: The psychodynamics of ecological debt'. In S. Weintrobe (ed.) *Engaging with Climate Change: Psychoanalytic and Interdisciplinary Perspectives*. Routledge.

2012: Dreams and play in child analysis today. In: Fonagy, P., Kachele, H., Leuzinger-Bohleber, M. and Taylor, D. (eds.) *The Significance of Dreams: Bridging Clinical and Extraclinical Research in Psychoanalysis*. Karnac.

2012: (with Michael Rustin) Fantasy and reality in Myazaki's animated world. *Psychoanalysis, Culture and Society*, 17 (2): 169–184.

2013: Finding out where and who one is: the special complexity of migration for adolescents. In A. Varchevker and E. McGinley (eds.) *Enduring Migration through the Life Cycle*. Karnac.

2013: (with S. M. G. Adamo and C. F. Pantaleo) An outsider in the nursery. *Infant Observation*, 16 (3): 230–243.

2014: The relevance of infant observation for early intervention: containment in theory and practice. *Infant Observation*, 17 (2): 97–114.

2016: A brief comment on Meltzer's approach to sexuality. *International Journal of Psychoanalysis*, 97 (3): 967–968.

2016: Doing things differently: an appreciation of Meltzer's contribution. *Journal of Child Psychotherapy*, 42 (11): 4–17.

2016: Infant observation. In A. Elliott and J. Prager (eds.) *The Routledge Handbook of Psychoanalysis in the Social Sciences and Humanities*. Routledge.

2016: Some comments on 'The absent object' by Edna O'Shaughnessy. *Journal of Child Psychotherapy*, 42 (2): 217–221.

2017: Creative responses to compromised beginnings in life: how to support families struggling with early difficulties. *Infant Observation*, 20 (2–3): 148–160.

2018: Psychoanalytic work with an adopted child with a history of early abuse and neglect. In P. Garvey and K. Long (eds.) *The Klein Tradition: Lines of Development – Evolution of Theory and Practice over the Decades.* Routledge.

2018: (with Michael Rustin) Work discussion presentations at the Vienna Conference in June 2016: introduction to the presentations. *Infant Observation*, 21 (2): 174–188.

2019: The inspiration of the ancients: the myth of Narcissus and Echo. *Infant Observation*, 22 (2–3): 86–91.

2020: Extending the reach of the 'talking cure'. In M. Waddell and S. Kraemer (eds.) *The Tavistock Century: 2020 Vision.* Phoenix.

Index

For Product Safety Concerns and Information please contact our EU
representative GPSR@taylorandfrancis.com
Taylor & Francis Verlag GmbH, Kaufingerstraße 24, 80331 München, Germany

www.ingramcontent.com/pod-product-compliance
Lightning Source LLC
Chambersburg PA
CBHW060240220326
41598CB00027B/3998